Hidden Healing Secrets of the Scriptures

Rediscovering God's Healing
Blueprint for Your Modern Life

The Hidden Architecture

He sent out his word and healed them; he rescued them from the grave.
Psalm 107:20

Table of Contents

Introduction: Rediscovering God's Blueprint for Healing

The Forgotten Wisdom of Scripture in Modern Times

Modern life moves at a pace unimaginable to those who lived in biblical times. We have constant access to information, yet we often feel more disconnected, stressed, and unwell than any generation before us. As we chase new wellness trends and quick fixes, it is easy to overlook the profound guidance that has been preserved in the very pages of Scripture — guidance that shaped the lives of entire communities for centuries. This forgotten wisdom is not about ancient rituals for their own sake, but about patterns God designed for human flourishing that remain as relevant now as they were thousands of years ago.

Throughout the Bible, we find references to nourishment, rest, emotional restoration, and spiritual alignment. The people of Israel were instructed on what to eat, how to cleanse, when to work, and when to stop. They were taught how to forgive, how to release burdens, and how to approach God in prayer. These were not arbitrary commands but part of a holistic framework for living in harmony with both body and spirit. When examined closely, many of these practices reveal striking parallels with what modern research now confirms as essential for health and emotional balance.

The disconnect arises because modern culture tends to fragment life into compartments: physical health, mental health, spiritual life, work, and relationships. Scripture, on the other hand, integrates them. A person's diet was connected to their worship. Rest was an act of trust in God. Forgiveness was not only a spiritual directive but also a release of emotional weight. This integration was not a religious add-on; it was life itself. Ignoring this holistic view has left many people searching for meaning in their wellness journey, hopping from one fad to the next without understanding the deeper design behind wholeness.

Another reason this wisdom feels forgotten is that our perception of the Bible has changed. For some, it has become purely a spiritual text, separated from anything practical. Others have dismissed it entirely in favor of modern science or secular philosophies. Yet when we take time to read the Scriptures through the lens of everyday life, we discover that God's Word speaks not only to the soul's eternal destiny but also to the daily rhythms of living well. From the manna in the wilderness to the call for Sabbath rest, from the anointing with oils to the power of prayer, every page holds insights that address very real struggles we face today.

This book aims to bridge that gap. It does not suggest abandoning modern medicine or proven health practices. Instead, it invites readers to rediscover the harmony between ancient biblical principles and today's understanding of human well-being. By exploring these teachings, you will see how timeless truths about rest, nourishment, forgiveness, and spiritual focus can guide you toward a life of greater peace and vitality. Each chapter offers not only historical and scriptural insights but also practical steps for applying them in modern contexts, always respecting the boundaries of what these practices can and cannot do.

To appreciate why this wisdom matters so much today, it helps to understand the contrast between biblical rhythms and modern patterns. In ancient times, life was naturally cyclical — tied to seasons, communal worship, and the rhythms of the land. Work and rest followed divine instruction. Food came directly from the earth, unprocessed and nutrient-dense. Worship and daily life were inseparable. Modern life, in contrast, is dominated by constant activity, artificial food systems, and relentless stress. We have abundance but lack balance, knowledge but little wisdom.

This imbalance is at the heart of many physical and emotional struggles people face. Chronic fatigue, anxiety, inflammation, and burnout are often symptoms of living out of sync with natural and spiritual rhythms. Reconnecting with the wisdom of Scripture does not erase all hardship, but it restores a foundation on which healing and peace can grow. It shifts focus from chasing external fixes to cultivating alignment with God's design, which impacts every aspect of life.

Recognizing this disconnect opens the door to change. When we slow down enough to notice the patterns God has woven into Scripture, we begin to see that many of the solutions we are searching for have been within reach all along. The biblical call to rest, for example, is not simply about observing a religious ritual; it is a deliberate invitation to step out of endless striving and trust in God's provision. When honored, this rhythm offers more than physical relief — it restores clarity, strengthens relationships, and reduces the stress that silently erodes well-being.

The same can be said of biblical fasting. While often misunderstood as a purely spiritual exercise, fasting also allows the body to reset and recalibrate. Ancient believers may not have had the scientific terminology we do today, but they understood that there was a purifying power in stepping away from constant consumption. Modern research by physicians such as Dr. Jason Fung (2016) has highlighted how fasting can improve insulin sensitivity and reduce inflammation, findings that echo the wisdom practiced by communities thousands of years ago. This kind of harmony between scripture and science encourages us to revisit these disciplines not as relics of the past but as gifts still relevant to our lives.

Forgiveness offers another striking example of forgotten wisdom. Scripture repeatedly urges believers to release bitterness and choose grace, not only for the sake of spiritual obedience but for personal freedom. Studies by Dr. Everett Worthington (2015) have demonstrated that people who practice forgiveness experience lower stress levels and improved mental health. These findings confirm what the Bible has taught all along: harboring resentment burdens the heart and, over time, even the body. The act of forgiving liberates both parties, creating space for healing that transcends physical health.

This rediscovery is not about adopting every practice exactly as it appeared in ancient times. Cultural context matters, and some instructions were given to specific people in specific circumstances. The goal is to discern timeless principles — the underlying truths about how God designed humans to thrive — and apply them in ways that are faithful and practical today. This requires humility, prayer, and willingness to learn rather than forcing scripture to fit modern trends or personal preferences.

As we move deeper into this journey, it becomes clear that forgotten wisdom is often simple rather than complicated. God's instructions rarely demand elaborate systems or expensive solutions. They point to natural foods, intentional rest, heartfelt prayer, community support, and quiet trust. These are disciplines that do not depend on advanced technology or constant consumption but on willingness to live differently from the cultural norm. In a world that glorifies busyness and instant results, these practices feel countercultural yet profoundly restorative.

The chapters ahead will explore these principles one by one, grounding each in its biblical foundation and offering practical ways to integrate them into modern life. This is not about achieving perfection or checking off religious tasks but about realignment — learning to live in a way that honors both God and the body He created. It is about small, faithful shifts that accumulate into lasting transformation. The promise is not the absence of hardship but the presence of peace, clarity, and renewed strength that come from walking in step with divine wisdom.

Rediscovering this forgotten wisdom is more than a personal health journey; it is an act of stewardship. Caring for our bodies, nurturing our minds, and tending to our spirits are ways of honoring the Creator who gave us life. When we live according to His design, we not only experience greater well-being ourselves but also become better equipped to serve, love, and encourage those around us. This ripple effect is one of the most overlooked aspects of biblical healing: it is never just about the individual. It restores families, strengthens communities, and testifies to God's goodness in a world longing for hope.

Why Ancient Practices Still Speak to Today's Ailments

The ailments that trouble people today might seem uniquely modern, shaped by technology, processed food, and relentless schedules. Yet at their core, many of these struggles mirror the same human challenges faced thousands of years ago: anxiety about the future, weariness from toil, physical suffering, and spiritual disconnection. The remarkable thing about the Bible is that, despite being written in an entirely different era, its wisdom cuts through time and speaks directly to these recurring human needs. Ancient practices recorded in Scripture were not bound to one culture or century; they address the universal rhythms and imbalances that have always affected the human body and soul.

Take the concept of rest. In a society that glorifies constant productivity, many suffer from exhaustion and burnout without realizing that chronic fatigue impacts more than just physical energy. It clouds thinking, increases irritability, and weakens resilience. Scripture anticipated this reality by commanding rhythms of rest long before modern science understood the impact of stress hormones on the body. The Sabbath was not only a commandment but also a gift — a divine invitation to pause, reconnect, and be restored. Current research by Dr. Matthew Walker (2017) on sleep demonstrates how vital rest is for cognitive function, emotional stability, and long-term health, affirming what God embedded into His creation from the beginning.

Another example is the biblical practice of fasting. While modern diets often focus on appearance or weight management, fasting in Scripture carries deeper meaning: a posture of humility before God and a way to realign priorities. Interestingly, modern medicine has found that intermittent fasting can improve metabolic health, reduce inflammation, and even support cellular repair processes. This does not mean fasting is a cure-all, nor should it replace medical advice, but it reveals that God's instructions often have layers of wisdom — both spiritual and physical — that we are only beginning to understand.

Herbal remedies and sacred oils also remain relevant in surprising ways. Frankincense, myrrh, and olive oil were central to worship and healing rituals throughout the Bible. They symbolized consecration and purity, yet they also held practical value. Today, studies on essential compounds in frankincense, for instance, suggest calming properties and potential anti-inflammatory effects. While these findings must be approached with balance and discernment, they demonstrate that practices rooted in reverence for God's creation can harmonize with what modern science is uncovering.

What makes these ancient practices compelling is not just their physical benefits but their ability to address the whole person. Modern solutions often isolate symptoms, focusing on immediate relief rather than root causes. Scripture, however, consistently integrates body, mind, and spirit. Practices like prayer, forgiveness, and community fellowship are not limited to spiritual well-being; they shape emotional resilience and even influence physical health. This holistic view reflects a truth that science is slowly confirming: our thoughts, emotions, and relationships profoundly affect our physical condition.

For many readers, the challenge lies in bridging these principles into modern life. It can feel unrealistic to adopt rhythms from an agrarian, temple-centered culture in today's urban and digital world. Yet the underlying truths — rest for renewal, fasting for focus, forgiveness for freedom — remain timeless. What changes is not the wisdom itself but the way we apply it. This book aims to uncover those timeless principles and translate them into practical, realistic steps suited for life today, without distorting their original meaning or purpose.

Understanding why these practices endure requires recognizing their source. They were not man-made self-help strategies but divine instructions flowing from God's understanding of human nature. He designed the body and soul, so His commands reflect what we most need, even when we fail to recognize it. When approached with humility, these practices reconnect us to the Creator's intent and offer pathways to wholeness that modern methods alone often cannot provide.

Recognizing this connection between divine wisdom and enduring human needs also helps dismantle the belief that ancient practices are outdated or irrelevant. When viewed through the lens of purpose rather than culture, they become guiding principles adaptable to any time or place. For instance, the instruction to forgive is not bound to a particular century or ritual but to the human condition itself. Bitterness and resentment harm relationships and weigh heavily on the heart, regardless of whether someone lives in a first-century village or a modern city. Modern studies by Dr. Loren Toussaint (2012) highlight how people who practice forgiveness experience lower levels of depression and greater life satisfaction, reinforcing what Scripture has emphasized for centuries: forgiveness liberates both spirit and body.

This timelessness also applies to the principle of community. From the earliest chapters of Genesis to the teachings of the New Testament, human beings are portrayed as relational by design. Commands to gather, share burdens, and pray together are not mere social niceties but vital components of spiritual and emotional well-being. Today, as isolation and loneliness reach unprecedented levels, the biblical model of fellowship offers a profound remedy. Even secular research confirms this, showing that strong community ties contribute to longer lifespans and improved mental health. Such findings remind us that God's design for community was not incidental but essential.

Applying these practices in a contemporary context requires discernment and intentionality. It is not about replicating ancient customs exactly as they were but capturing their essence and purpose. Observing a Sabbath today might look different than in ancient Israel, yet the principle of pausing work and centering life on God remains equally transformative. Fasting may not follow the same patterns as it did in the wilderness or the temple, yet the heart posture of dependence and humility it fosters is as needed now as ever. What matters is staying rooted in biblical truth while allowing room for wise adaptation.

This understanding also counters the temptation to treat these practices as quick fixes. While they can bring significant benefits, they are not formulas for instant healing. They invite a process of alignment that unfolds over time, shaping habits, mindset, and priorities. This slower, more faithful approach contrasts sharply with the culture of instant gratification. It encourages patience and perseverance, virtues that deepen spiritual maturity and allow true transformation to take place gradually but profoundly.

Ultimately, the enduring relevance of these practices reveals something about God's character. He gave principles that transcend generations because He knows what His creation needs in every age. As technology and culture evolve, the human heart continues to wrestle with fear, pride, longing, and hope. God's solutions remain steady amid that change, offering an anchor when modern advice feels chaotic or contradictory. The practices He set in motion still whisper truth to restless hearts, pointing them back to rhythms that foster life rather than drain it.

By revisiting these ancient instructions with fresh eyes, we recover more than just health habits. We rediscover a way of living that draws us closer to the Creator and helps us navigate modern challenges with wisdom rather than confusion. The following chapters will unfold these principles in detail, inviting you to explore how rest, prayer, fasting, forgiveness, and other biblical rhythms can become part of your daily life. They will not replace the role of medical care or modern understanding, but they will offer a deeper foundation — one that restores meaning to the pursuit of well-being and points to the wholeness God intended from the beginning.

Healing as Restoration: What This Book Is (and Isn't)

When many people hear the word "healing," their minds immediately jump to the idea of a cure — a quick solution that removes discomfort and restores life to what it was before illness or hardship. While this is understandable, the biblical picture of healing is far broader and deeper. In Scripture, healing is rarely portrayed as a one-time event; it is often described as a process of restoration, reconciliation, and renewal. It is about being made whole in body, mind, and spirit, not merely about the absence of pain or disease.

This distinction is essential to understand from the beginning. The purpose of this book is not to promise miraculous cures or instant relief from serious conditions. It is not a substitute for medical care, nor does it claim to reveal hidden formulas that guarantee perfect health. Those kinds of promises are not only unrealistic but can be harmful, leaving people discouraged when their expectations are not met. Instead, the focus here is on uncovering biblical principles and rhythms that support overall well-being and help restore balance to areas of life that modern living has often thrown out of order.

In the Bible, restoration is closely tied to relationship — first with God, and then with others. Many of the ailments we struggle with today, from stress to loneliness to chronic fatigue, are deeply connected to disconnection. Disconnection from God's design for rest, disconnection from nourishing foods, disconnection from supportive community, and disconnection from the peace that comes with forgiveness. Healing, in this sense, is not about going back to an imagined ideal but about moving toward alignment with God's original intent for human flourishing.

This perspective changes how we approach the practices explored in this book. Prayer is not treated as a ritual to earn healing but as a means of drawing closer to the One who heals. Fasting is not about punishing the body but about simplifying life to listen more deeply to God's voice. Observing rhythms of rest, such as the Sabbath, is not about legalism but about trusting that we do not have to live enslaved to constant productivity. These practices are spiritual at their core, yet they also bring

15

tangible benefits to mental and physical health. The beauty lies in how seamlessly they integrate both realms.

Understanding what this book is not will help guard against common misunderstandings. It is not a manual for replacing professional care with spiritual disciplines. God often works through skilled doctors, counselors, and nutritionists. Scripture itself recognizes the value of practical wisdom and community support in times of illness or hardship. What this book offers is complementary: it invites you to explore how spiritual practices can nurture resilience, peace, and vitality alongside whatever other steps you may be taking for your health.

By framing healing as restoration, we also create space for grace. Some struggles may not resolve in the way we hope, yet even in ongoing challenges, the journey of drawing closer to God can bring profound renewal. Many biblical figures experienced God's presence and peace amid trials rather than through their immediate removal. The Apostle Paul, for instance, spoke of a "thorn in the flesh" that remained despite his prayers for relief, yet it became a source of deeper dependence on God's strength. This reminds us that healing is not always about changing circumstances but about transformation within them.

Recognizing this broader view of healing prepares us for a more realistic and hopeful journey. It shifts expectations away from instant fixes toward sustainable change and spiritual growth. It also opens the door to appreciating the small but meaningful shifts that come with living in harmony with God's design: clearer thinking, lighter emotional burdens, deeper rest, and a greater sense of purpose. These changes, though subtle at first, can ripple into every area of life, from relationships to physical health.

Seeing healing through the lens of restoration also encourages a more holistic approach. It prompts us to consider how our thoughts, choices, and environments contribute to the health of our entire being. A person may seek physical relief from fatigue, but deeper examination might reveal patterns of anxiety, unresolved conflict, or neglect of rest that are equally demanding attention. By tending to these interconnected layers, healing becomes more than symptom management. It becomes an invitation to reorient life around principles that bring lasting peace.

This journey is not passive. Scripture often depicts healing as involving active participation — steps of obedience, faith, and intentional living. Naaman, the Syrian commander healed of leprosy, had to wash himself in the Jordan River seven times as instructed by the prophet Elisha. The man born blind in the Gospel of John was told to go and wash in the Pool of Siloam. These stories remind us that while God is the ultimate source of healing, He often invites His people into partnership, calling them to trust and act even when they do not fully understand the outcome.

In practical terms, this partnership may look like creating space for prayer when life feels too busy, choosing whole foods that honor the body's design, or seeking reconciliation in strained relationships. It may mean observing rhythms of rest, fasting with intention, or embracing simplicity in a culture of excess. These small shifts, grounded in biblical truth, gradually reestablish balance and allow God's peace to permeate daily life. They are not about earning healing but about aligning with the Creator's wisdom.

Holding this perspective also guards against disappointment when outcomes differ from expectations. If healing is defined narrowly as the removal of every struggle, anything less can feel like failure. But when healing is understood as restoration of wholeness — body, mind, and spirit — progress can be recognized in many forms: greater resilience, deeper faith, renewed joy, or restored relationships. These fruits are as much a part of healing as physical relief, and they often have a more enduring impact.

This approach respects the complexity of human experience. Some conditions may improve quickly, while others may persist for reasons we cannot fully understand. Yet even in ongoing difficulty, God's presence and promises remain steady. The Psalms, filled with raw honesty about suffering, continually return to trust in God's goodness and sustaining power. They remind us that restoration often unfolds in stages, sometimes quietly, as we continue walking with Him.

By clarifying what this book is and is not, the path forward becomes clearer. The chapters ahead will explore specific biblical practices — from fasting and prayer to forgiveness and Sabbath rest — with both reverence and practicality. Each principle will be rooted in scripture, illuminated by context, and translated into actionable steps suitable for modern life. At every stage, the emphasis will remain on wholeness rather than quick fixes, on alignment with God's design rather than self-reliance.

Approaching healing this way also cultivates humility. It shifts the focus from striving for control to trusting the One who knows us fully and cares for every detail of our lives. This posture of trust allows room for both gratitude and growth, even in seasons of uncertainty. It is in this space that true restoration begins — a quiet yet profound transformation that touches body, renews mind, and draws the soul closer to the heart of God.

Part I. Foundations of Biblical Healing

Every meaningful journey begins with understanding where you stand and where you are headed. Before diving into specific practices like fasting, rest, or prayer, it is vital to explore the foundations of why these practices matter in the first place. Scripture presents a vision of human life that is far richer than what most people experience day to day — a vision rooted in wholeness, harmony, and a close relationship with God. This first part lays that groundwork, helping you see healing not as an isolated event but as part of a larger story that has been unfolding since creation.

The Bible begins with a picture of perfect alignment. In the Garden of Eden, there was no division between body and spirit, no stress or striving, no fractured relationships. The food was abundant and natural, work was purposeful but not exhausting, and God's presence was near. That blueprint remains at the core of God's design for human flourishing. Yet through disobedience and separation from Him, that harmony was disrupted, and the consequences — sickness, anxiety, brokenness — entered the human story.

Understanding this contrast between God's original intent and humanity's current struggles is the starting point for restoration. Healing, in the biblical sense, is about returning to that divine pattern. It is about rediscovering the rhythms of living that honor both the Creator and the creation. This is not about recreating a primitive lifestyle but about realigning with principles that have proven timeless: nourishing the body as God intended, resting in His care, and integrating faith into every aspect of life.

For the reader searching for relief from stress, fatigue, or a sense of spiritual distance, these truths are not abstract theology. They offer a practical way forward. When viewed through the lens of Scripture, everyday choices — what we eat, how we rest, how we handle conflict

— become opportunities to live closer to God's design. This part of the book will guide you into that framework, showing how foundational principles like creation, diet, and alignment with God's wisdom set the stage for deeper transformation in the chapters ahead.

Chapter 1: God's Design for the Human Body

The Creation Blueprint: Fearfully and Wonderfully Made

Long before modern medicine mapped the human genome or explored the complexities of the nervous system, Scripture declared a profound truth: human beings are "fearfully and wonderfully made" (Psalm 139:14). This verse, often quoted in moments of personal affirmation, carries a depth that goes far beyond poetic comfort. It points to intentional design — a Creator who shaped every cell, every system, every rhythm of life with purpose and care. To understand biblical healing, we must first understand this foundational truth: our bodies and souls were designed with harmony in mind.

In the opening chapters of Genesis, we see humanity placed in an environment perfectly suited for flourishing. The garden provided nourishment in abundance, meaningful work, beauty to behold, and uninterrupted fellowship with God. Nothing in that setting was accidental. The human body was formed from the dust of the earth yet infused with divine breath, a union of physical and spiritual that reflects the Creator's intent for wholeness. This blueprint is not simply historical; it is a mirror for what health, in its truest sense, was always meant to be.

Acknowledging this design reshapes how we view ourselves. Many people today carry frustration toward their bodies, seeing them as sources of pain or disappointment. Cultural messages about perfection and appearance only deepen this sense of dissatisfaction. Yet the biblical perspective invites reverence rather than resentment. To be "fearfully" made is to be created with awe-inspiring intricacy, and to be "wonderfully" made is to be imbued with inherent worth. Every heartbeat, every breath, every intricate process happening beneath the surface is a testament to divine craftsmanship.

Modern science continues to uncover layers of complexity that affirm this truth. The immune system alone — constantly scanning, repairing, and defending — functions with remarkable precision. The body's capacity for healing wounds, regenerating cells, and adapting to challenges demonstrates wisdom woven into creation itself. Rather than viewing health as something to achieve through sheer willpower, recognizing this inherent design invites us to steward what has already been given. Stewardship begins with respect: treating the body not as disposable but as a sacred vessel entrusted to our care.

This view also reframes the purpose of biblical practices discussed throughout this book. Sabbath rest, fasting, prayer, and forgiveness are not arbitrary commands meant to burden us; they are rhythms designed to keep body and spirit aligned. Ignoring them does not only affect spiritual life — it impacts physical and emotional well-being. When we neglect rest, overload ourselves with stress, or carry bitterness, we disrupt the balance God intended. Conversely, when we embrace His rhythms, we cooperate with the natural design already present within us. Seeing ourselves as part of God's creation also calls for humility. While modern advancements in health and medicine are blessings, they can lead to an illusion of control. The biblical blueprint reminds us that ultimate wisdom belongs to the Creator, and true wholeness flows from living in harmony with His design. This is not a rejection of science but an acknowledgment that the deepest answers to human flourishing are spiritual as well as physical.

Understanding this foundation prepares us for what follows: exploring how specific biblical principles can restore balance to modern life. Each principle builds on the recognition that we are more than physical bodies and more than spiritual souls — we are integrated beings designed for connection with God, others, and creation itself. Grasping this truth is the first step toward the restoration the Bible envisions.

This understanding of being intricately designed also highlights the responsibility that comes with it. Caring for the body is not only a matter of personal health but of honoring the Creator. Scripture speaks of the body as a temple of the Holy Spirit, a dwelling place for God's presence. When we see our bodies through this lens, every choice — what we eat, how we rest, the way we handle stress — becomes an act of stewardship rather than a burden of self-improvement. It shifts motivation from appearance or performance to reverence and gratitude.

Recognizing God's design can also reshape how we view our limitations. Many people wrestle with shame over illness, weakness, or fatigue, believing these struggles diminish their worth. Yet Scripture consistently affirms dignity regardless of physical condition. The image of God imprinted on humanity is not erased by illness or imperfection. This perspective is freeing because it allows healing to be understood not only as physical recovery but as restoration of peace, identity, and purpose. Even in times when the body does not function as we wish, we can live from a place of wholeness grounded in God's truth.

Practical reflection on this blueprint invites us to examine daily rhythms. Are we aligning with the natural cycles God established — periods of activity balanced with rest, nourishment drawn from whole foods, moments of stillness woven into busy schedules? Modern life often pulls us away from these patterns. Constant stimulation, processed diets, and relentless stress work against the harmony our bodies were designed to thrive in. Reintegrating biblical practices into daily life is not about recreating the past but about reclaiming principles that still meet our deepest needs.

Scientific insights can deepen appreciation for these rhythms without diminishing their spiritual meaning. For example, research by Dr. Herbert Benson (2000) on the "relaxation response" shows how intentional rest and prayerful meditation lower stress hormones and support cardiovascular health. These findings echo what Scripture has long taught about the renewing power of stillness before God. They also remind us that spiritual disciplines are not disconnected from physical health; they work together, reflecting the integrated nature of human design.

Approaching the body as part of God's masterpiece leads to a more compassionate relationship with ourselves. Instead of striving for unrealistic ideals, we can focus on caring for what has been entrusted to us. This does not mean ignoring areas where improvement is needed but approaching change with patience and gratitude. It means listening to the signals our bodies give us — fatigue, tension, even cravings — and responding with wisdom rather than guilt or neglect.

This foundation sets the tone for the chapters that follow. As we explore fasting, prayer, forgiveness, and Sabbath rest, we will return repeatedly to this central truth: the God who designed us knows what we need. His instructions are not arbitrary rules but pathways to restore what has been lost in a culture of hurry and disconnection. Accepting that we are fearfully and wonderfully made is more than acknowledging beauty in creation; it is an invitation to live in alignment with the One who formed us, finding healing not just in the absence of illness but in the presence of wholeness.

How Sin and Stress Distort God's Original Plan

The harmony of creation described in Genesis did not remain intact for long. Through disobedience, humanity stepped out of alignment with God's design, and the consequences rippled through every aspect of life. Sin introduced separation — from God, from one another, and from the wholeness that was originally built into the human experience. This separation affected not only spiritual connection but also physical health and emotional well-being. The Bible's narrative of brokenness helps explain why the world today often feels so fragmented and why so many struggle with ailments that extend far beyond the physical.

When sin entered the picture, so did stress in its most fundamental form. The immediate reaction of Adam and Eve after eating from the forbidden tree was fear and shame. They hid from God, covered themselves, and felt exposed. This pattern of anxiety, guilt, and self-protection has echoed through human history ever since. It is more than a theological concept; it is something we feel in our bodies. Elevated heart rate, shallow breathing, and tense muscles are physical signs of the same disconnection described in those early chapters of Scripture.

Stress, in a broader sense, reflects the strain of living in a world no longer operating as God intended. While not all stress is inherently bad — short-term stress can motivate action and protect from danger — chronic stress undermines health and relationships. Modern research confirms what Scripture implies: prolonged anxiety and tension weaken the immune system, disrupt sleep, and contribute to conditions like heart disease and depression. Dr. Bruce McEwen's work in neuroendocrinology (1998) identified how ongoing stress reshapes the brain's architecture, affecting memory, mood, and decision-making. These insights mirror biblical warnings about the heavy toll of worry and fear on the human heart.

Beyond its physiological impact, stress compounds the effects of sin by influencing behavior. People under constant pressure are more likely to make unhealthy choices, from poor eating habits to neglecting rest or relationships. In Scripture, this cycle is evident: when people turned from God's guidance, chaos followed, often leading to destructive decisions

25

that worsened their struggles. Modern life continues this pattern. The relentless pace of work, the pressure to achieve, and the constant noise of digital distractions leave little room for reflection, prayer, or connection with others.

Sin also distorts the way people view themselves. Instead of seeing themselves as image-bearers of God, many view themselves through the lens of inadequacy or comparison. This distorted identity fuels further stress, creating a loop that is difficult to break. The pursuit of worth through performance, appearance, or material success becomes exhausting, yet never fully satisfies. Biblical narratives repeatedly highlight this tension, showing how humanity's attempts to find fulfillment apart from God lead to restlessness rather than peace.

Understanding how sin and stress distort God's original plan is not meant to condemn but to clarify why restoration is necessary. Recognizing the source of the problem points us toward the solution. If separation brought disorder, then reconciliation brings healing. If misplaced priorities fueled anxiety, returning to God's rhythms offers relief. This shift in perspective prepares us to explore how biblical practices can serve as pathways back to balance and wholeness.

Acknowledging the ways sin and stress disrupt life also reveals why so many modern solutions feel incomplete. People often attempt to address symptoms — sleeplessness, anxiety, poor health — without addressing the deeper fractures beneath them. Diet changes or stress management techniques can bring temporary relief, but without addressing the spiritual disconnection at the root, lasting peace remains elusive. Scripture repeatedly calls people back to the source of true rest, not simply to escape hardship but to be restored to relationship with the One who created them.

This understanding reframes what healing looks like in practical terms. Restoring balance involves more than simply removing stressors; it requires reordering priorities around God's wisdom. Jesus Himself highlighted this when He invited the weary and burdened to come to Him for rest, promising a yoke that is easy and a burden that is light. This invitation is not passive. It requires choosing to step away from the constant demands of culture and trusting that God's provision is enough, even when circumstances remain challenging.

Recognizing the role of stress in modern life also offers an opportunity for compassion — both toward ourselves and others. Many carry unacknowledged burdens that shape their health and relationships. Extending grace in these moments aligns with the character of Christ, who consistently met people in their brokenness with understanding rather than condemnation. This posture opens the door to genuine transformation, as people feel safe to release guilt and begin the work of realignment.

Modern research provides additional insight into how this process unfolds in the body. Studies by Dr. Robert Sapolsky (2004) on stress hormones, particularly cortisol, show how prolonged stress affects nearly every system: immune function, digestion, cardiovascular health, and even memory. These findings echo biblical principles that warn against worry and call believers to cast their anxieties on God. When we live in a state of constant tension, the body pays the price, but when we cultivate trust and rest, healing mechanisms that God built into our design begin to function as intended.

Understanding this connection between spiritual and physical realities creates space for hope. Healing is not about erasing every trace of stress or avoiding all hardship, which is impossible in a fallen world. It is about learning to live differently within those realities — shifting from self-reliance to God-dependence, from chaos to rhythms of peace, from fragmented priorities to integrated living. Each step in this process draws us closer to the life God envisioned, even when challenges remain.

As we move forward, the biblical practices explored in the coming chapters will offer concrete ways to begin this realignment. Fasting, prayer, forgiveness, and rest are not isolated rituals but parts of a larger framework designed to counteract the distortions introduced by sin and sustained by chronic stress. When embraced with humility and consistency, these practices help restore the harmony that was present in the beginning — a harmony that is still available to those willing to return to the Creator's blueprint for life.

Aligning Modern Habits with Biblical Principles

Modern life is filled with habits that most people never stop to question. From the way we eat to how we work, rest, and connect with others, daily routines are often shaped by convenience rather than intentional design. Yet when we compare these patterns to the principles laid out in Scripture, we discover significant gaps. The Bible describes a rhythm of life centered on trust in God, balance between work and rest, and care for both body and soul. Bringing our habits into alignment with these principles is not about rigid rules but about rediscovering a way of living that leads to wholeness.

One of the most striking contrasts between biblical living and modern habits is pace. Scripture reveals a God who established seasons and rhythms: six days of work followed by a day of rest, times of fasting balanced by times of feasting, moments of solitude balanced by community gatherings. In today's culture, constant activity has replaced these cycles. Work bleeds into evenings and weekends, technology keeps us perpetually "on," and rest feels like an indulgence rather than a necessity. This shift contributes to chronic stress, exhaustion, and disconnection from God and others.

Realigning our pace begins with acknowledging the value of rest as a spiritual and physical need. The Sabbath principle is not simply about ceasing labor but about trusting that we do not hold the world together by our effort. Setting aside time to stop, reflect, and reconnect with God restores perspective and allows the body to recover from the relentless demands of daily life. Modern studies on rest and recovery, such as the work of Dr. Matthew Walker (2017), confirm that regular restorative sleep and downtime significantly improve cognitive function and emotional health, aligning with what Scripture has long taught.

Diet is another area where modern habits often diverge from biblical wisdom. The biblical narrative frequently highlights foods in their natural form — fruits, grains, fish, and clean meats — and emphasizes moderation and gratitude. Today's food systems, however, prioritize speed and shelf life, leading to processed options that disconnect us from the nourishment God originally intended. Aligning dietary habits with biblical principles does not require adopting a specific ancient diet but involves choosing foods that honor the body's design and foster energy and clarity rather than depletion.

Technology introduces additional challenges. While tools like smartphones and social media can be beneficial, they often distract from deeper relationships and quiet moments with God. The constant noise of modern life competes with the stillness needed for prayer and reflection. Scripture repeatedly calls for intentional quiet — times when God's voice can be heard above the clamor of daily life. Creating boundaries around technology, such as designated unplugged times, can help cultivate this kind of sacred space.

Aligning modern habits with biblical principles also involves rethinking how we handle stress and emotional burdens. Instead of carrying anxiety alone or numbing it through unhealthy coping mechanisms, Scripture invites us to cast our cares on God and seek community support. This shift requires humility, as it involves admitting need and trusting in God's provision rather than relying solely on personal strength. It is a countercultural move in a world that celebrates self-sufficiency, yet it is central to living in alignment with the Creator's design.

Making these adjustments requires intentional reflection on the habits that dominate daily life. Many are so ingrained that they happen automatically: checking messages first thing in the morning, eating hurried meals without gratitude, multitasking through prayer, or filling every spare moment with noise. Realignment begins with awareness. Taking time to notice how these patterns affect physical energy, emotional balance, and spiritual focus reveals where change is most needed. This kind of honest self-examination reflects the biblical call to "consider your ways" and invites God to shine light on areas that have drifted from His design.

Small, deliberate shifts often create the most sustainable change. For someone struggling with constant hurry, this might mean carving out a short period each day for quiet reflection or prayer before the demands of work begin. For another, it could involve introducing a weekly family meal where gratitude is expressed and distractions are set aside. Over time, these rhythms cultivate a deeper sense of peace and connection.

They also build resilience, allowing a person to face challenges from a place of spiritual grounding rather than constant reaction.

Modern research affirms the benefits of these shifts without diminishing their spiritual value. For instance, studies by Dr. Kristin Neff (2011) on self-compassion highlight how gentle awareness of personal shortcomings reduces stress and supports healthier behavior change. This aligns closely with the biblical principle of grace — approaching growth not from shame but from a desire to honor God and steward what He has entrusted to us. Integrating scientific insights with scriptural wisdom demonstrates how faith and evidence can work together to guide practical transformation.

An important part of aligning habits with biblical principles is recognizing that this is not about perfection. Scripture consistently portrays God's people as works in progress, learning to trust Him step by step. The aim is not to meet an unattainable standard but to live more intentionally, inviting God into choices that shape health and relationships. Even small adjustments, when made consistently, can yield profound shifts in outlook and energy. These incremental changes are often how deep restoration unfolds.

This realignment also fosters a different perspective on success. Modern culture often measures achievement by productivity, appearance, or material gain, but biblical principles redefine success as faithfulness, love, and stewardship. When habits begin to reflect this perspective, life becomes less about striving and more about living in harmony with God's presence. This shift offers relief from the pressures of comparison and competition, replacing them with contentment and purpose.

As the chapters ahead explore specific practices like fasting, prayer, forgiveness, and Sabbath rest, they will provide detailed guidance on how to integrate these rhythms into daily life without overwhelming schedules or unrealistic demands. The goal is to build habits that nurture both body and spirit, anchored in the conviction that God's design leads to true flourishing. By gradually aligning modern routines with these timeless principles, a life marked by peace, clarity, and renewed strength becomes not only possible but sustainable.

Chapter 2: Food as Sacred Fuel

The Eden Diet: What Scripture Reveals About Nourishment

At the very beginning of the biblical story, before laws were given or sacrifices were established, God addressed one of humanity's most basic needs: nourishment. In the Garden of Eden, food was abundant, natural, and freely provided. Genesis 1:29 records God's words to Adam and Eve: "I give you every seed-bearing plant on the face of the whole earth and every tree that has fruit with seed in it. They will be yours for food." This verse is more than a historical detail; it offers a glimpse into God's original intention for how humans were meant to fuel their bodies.

The Eden narrative presents a vision of eating that is strikingly different from modern habits. Food was not about indulgence or restriction but about sustenance and gratitude. It came directly from creation, unprocessed and rich with nutrients. The first humans did not count calories, chase fad diets, or view food as an enemy to be controlled. Instead, nourishment was integrated seamlessly into life, reflecting trust in the Creator's provision. This perspective is still relevant, especially in a culture where eating is often driven by convenience, emotion, or marketing rather than true hunger or intentional care for the body.

Looking closely at the Eden diet reveals several principles that can guide modern choices. First is the emphasis on plant-based foods — fruits, grains, nuts, and seeds. While Scripture does not mandate vegetarianism for all, it highlights the richness and sufficiency of these foods as foundational for health. Later passages in the Bible, including the dietary allowances given after the flood, expand the variety of what people may eat, but the principle of simplicity and natural provision remains consistent. These foods, abundant in vitamins, fiber, and essential fats, align closely with what contemporary nutrition science recognizes as beneficial for long-term health.

The Eden account also underscores the idea of stewardship. God placed Adam and Eve in the garden "to work it and take care of it" (Genesis

2:15). This implies responsibility not only for the land but also for how its produce is used. Nourishment in God's design is never purely about the individual; it is connected to community and creation care. Choosing foods that honor the body and respect the resources provided reflects a posture of gratitude and humility rather than exploitation.

Another key element in this biblical picture is the role of gratitude. Food in Eden was received as a gift, not taken for granted or hoarded. Modern eating patterns often strip meals of this sense of sacredness, reducing them to hurried moments or mindless consumption. Reintroducing gratitude — pausing to give thanks before eating, acknowledging God as the source — transforms a basic necessity into an act of worship. It also cultivates mindfulness, helping us listen to our bodies and eat with greater awareness.

Understanding the Eden diet does not mean attempting to replicate it exactly, which would be impractical and unnecessary. The goal is to extract timeless principles that can inform our choices today. Natural foods, moderation, gratitude, and respect for God's provision form a framework for eating that promotes both health and spiritual alignment. When we begin to view food through this lens, it ceases to be a source of guilt or confusion and becomes an avenue for living in harmony with God's original plan.

This framework also invites us to reconsider the emotional relationship many people have with food. In the modern world, eating often becomes a response to stress, boredom, or celebration, rather than a mindful act of nourishment. The biblical view calls for a return to intention. When we see food as part of God's good creation, every meal becomes an opportunity to honor Him, rather than a source of conflict or overindulgence. This shift does not require rigid rules but fosters a deeper sense of awareness and balance.

Applying these principles also challenges the culture of excess that dominates much of today's food environment. Processed snacks, oversized portions, and constant access to sugary drinks would have been unthinkable in biblical times. Returning to simpler, more natural foods can help restore balance not only to physical health but also to the way we relate to God's gifts. This does not mean rejecting all modern conveniences but approaching them with discernment. A meal prepared from fresh ingredients and eaten with gratitude aligns far more closely with biblical nourishment than the hurried consumption of highly processed foods.

Scientific research adds an additional layer of confirmation to these ancient principles. Studies by Dr. Walter Willett at Harvard (2013) have consistently shown that diets rich in fruits, vegetables, whole grains, and healthy fats reduce the risk of chronic disease and support longevity. These findings mirror the abundance of plant-based foods emphasized in Genesis and demonstrate how modern understanding continues to validate God's original provision. When approached with humility, this harmony between faith and science can strengthen trust in Scripture's relevance for everyday life.

Another overlooked element of the Eden narrative is moderation. The garden was filled with variety, yet there were boundaries. Adam and Eve were free to eat from every tree except one, a reminder that freedom and restraint must coexist. This principle speaks powerfully to modern struggles with overconsumption. Learning to recognize sufficiency — to enjoy what is provided without constant craving for more — fosters contentment and guards against the physical and emotional strain of excess.

Integrating these insights into modern life begins with small, practical steps. Choosing whole foods more often, slowing down to give thanks before meals, and eating until satisfied rather than overfull are simple yet profound ways to realign habits with biblical principles. Over time, these practices not only improve physical health but also nurture gratitude and trust in God's care. They remind us that eating is not separate from spiritual life; it is one of the most consistent opportunities we have to live out our faith in daily routines.

Ultimately, the Eden diet invites us into a deeper relationship with both creation and the Creator. It teaches that the food we eat carries meaning beyond calories and nutrients. It reflects God's generosity and calls us to respond with gratitude, stewardship, and humility. By returning to these timeless principles, we move closer to the harmony God intended — a way of eating that nourishes body and soul and reminds us daily of the One who provides.

Clean vs. Unclean Foods: Lessons Beyond the Law

When reading through the Old Testament, few topics spark as much curiosity as the dietary laws given to Israel. Leviticus 11 and Deuteronomy 14 describe in detail which animals were considered clean and permissible to eat and which were unclean and forbidden. These distinctions shaped the daily lives of God's people, influencing what they farmed, hunted, prepared, and shared at their tables. For modern readers, these laws can seem distant, even irrelevant, yet they hold enduring lessons about God's care for His people and the principles that guide healthy, intentional living.

To understand these instructions, it is important to see them within their covenantal context. The clean and unclean food laws were not arbitrary restrictions. They were part of a larger system that set Israel apart as a holy people, distinct from surrounding nations. Holiness in this sense meant more than moral purity; it encompassed every aspect of life, including what was eaten. God's call to be holy as He is holy was woven into daily routines, reminding the Israelites constantly of their identity and dependence on Him.

The reasons behind these distinctions have been debated for centuries. Some scholars see them as primarily symbolic, pointing to deeper spiritual truths about purity and obedience. Others note practical health benefits, observing that many of the prohibited animals were more likely to carry disease or spoil quickly in the climate and conditions of the ancient Near East. While the Bible does not explicitly give a single explanation, both perspectives highlight a key principle: God's commands are always given for the good of His people, whether their purposes are immediately understood or not.

For Christians today, the question naturally arises: Are these dietary laws still binding? The New Testament provides clarity. In passages like Mark 7:19 and Acts 10, we see Jesus and later Peter declaring all foods clean, signaling a shift from ritual purity laws to the deeper call of heart transformation. The Apostle Paul reinforces this in Romans 14 and 1 Corinthians 8, teaching that food itself does not make someone righteous or unrighteous before God, though believers should exercise wisdom and sensitivity in their choices.

This does not mean, however, that the concept of clean and unclean has nothing to teach us. The heart of the matter lies not in rigid adherence to dietary restrictions but in the principles underlying them. The clean/unclean distinction reminds us that what we consume matters, both physically and spiritually. Food is not morally neutral; it can either support or hinder our well-being and clarity of mind. In a culture where eating is often divorced from any sense of spiritual significance, this perspective challenges us to be more intentional.

The principle of discernment is central to applying these lessons today. While the ritual laws no longer define holiness, the call to approach food with wisdom and gratitude remains. Many modern health struggles stem from eating habits that ignore the body's design, relying heavily on processed foods, excessive sugars, and artificial ingredients. By contrast, the biblical pattern emphasizes simplicity, moderation, and attentiveness to what truly nourishes. When we view eating as stewardship rather than indulgence, our choices begin to reflect both reverence for God and care for ourselves.

An important takeaway from the clean and unclean distinctions is the idea that not everything available is beneficial. The Apostle Paul echoes this principle in 1 Corinthians 10:23, writing, "I have the right to do anything," but clarifying that "not everything is beneficial." This perspective is vital in a world of overwhelming food options. While believers are free from the ritual obligations of the Old Covenant, freedom does not eliminate responsibility. Choosing foods that align with God's design for the body supports clarity of mind, energy for service, and resilience in daily life.

Modern research often affirms these underlying principles, even without referencing Scripture. For example, studies by Dr. Michael Greger (2015) highlight the health risks associated with diets high in processed meats and refined sugars, while emphasizing the benefits of whole, plant-rich foods for reducing chronic disease. Although these findings are rooted in scientific observation rather than theological teaching, they harmonize with the scriptural call to honor the body through mindful nourishment.

Beyond physical health, the clean and unclean framework carries spiritual significance. It invites us to pause before eating, to acknowledge that food is not just fuel but part of God's provision. This mindfulness transforms mealtime into an opportunity for gratitude and reflection. It also cultivates self-control, a fruit of the Spirit that extends far beyond diet into every aspect of life. By practicing restraint at the table, we learn habits of discipline that shape how we approach work, relationships, and spiritual growth.

Practical application does not require adopting ancient dietary restrictions. Instead, it calls for adopting the wisdom behind them: choosing foods that promote life rather than deplete it, recognizing boundaries that protect rather than confine, and cultivating gratitude in the ordinary act of eating. This approach bridges the gap between ancient text and modern context, allowing believers to honor God without falling into legalism.

Ultimately, the lesson of clean and unclean foods points toward a larger reality. Holiness was never meant to be confined to diet alone but to permeate the entire life of God's people. What we eat can reflect that holiness, not by following strict rules, but by approaching nourishment as part of our worship and stewardship. In doing so, even the simplest meal becomes a reminder of God's care and an opportunity to live in alignment with His design.

Practical Biblical Meal Frameworks for Today

Applying biblical principles to daily meals can feel challenging in a world where convenience and speed often dictate what ends up on our plates. Yet Scripture offers a framework that is not about rigid rules but about aligning food choices with God's design for nourishment, balance, and gratitude. Translating these timeless truths into modern routines allows us to move from theory to practice, creating meals that support both health and spiritual well-being.

The starting point is to view food as part of a bigger picture. In biblical times, meals were rarely rushed. They were occasions for connection, gratitude, and remembrance of God's provision. Bread was broken and shared, prayers were spoken aloud, and the act of eating was deeply relational. Bringing even a portion of this posture into modern life can transform meals from hurried refueling stops into opportunities for mindfulness and worship. This perspective does not require elaborate preparations but rather a shift in attitude — slowing down enough to give thanks and to recognize that every bite is a gift.

A second principle drawn from Scripture is simplicity. The foods mentioned in the Bible are generally whole and minimally processed: grains, fruits, vegetables, legumes, fish, and clean meats. This does not mean recreating ancient diets exactly but embracing the concept of foods that are as close to their natural form as possible. When we focus on whole foods, we naturally reduce our intake of additives, excess sugars, and preservatives that dominate much of modern eating. This shift aligns not only with biblical wisdom but also with modern nutritional science, which consistently links whole-food diets to better health outcomes and lower rates of chronic disease.

Portion and balance are also key elements of a biblical meal framework. While the Bible celebrates abundance, it also warns against gluttony and overindulgence. Meals were meant to satisfy, not to overwhelm. Moderation allows us to enjoy food fully without falling into extremes of either deprivation or excess. This principle is particularly relevant today, where oversized portions and constant snacking can lead to fatigue and imbalances that affect physical and emotional health.

Choosing portions that meet needs without excess fosters both gratitude and self-control.

Building meals around these principles can also provide clarity amid the confusion of modern dietary trends. Instead of chasing every new fad, grounding choices in simple biblical wisdom offers stability. A meal that includes a variety of colorful vegetables, a source of clean protein, whole grains, and healthy fats reflects the balance God intended. When paired with mindful eating and gratitude, this approach nourishes more than the body; it nurtures contentment and peace of mind.

These frameworks also encourage adaptability. The Bible's teachings on food were given across diverse times and settings — from the wilderness to fertile farmlands, from scarcity to abundance. This flexibility reminds us that biblical principles can be applied in any culture or circumstance. Whether preparing a simple meal at home or making thoughtful choices while traveling, the goal remains the same: honoring God through what we eat and how we approach the act of eating itself.

Practical application begins with assessing what is already present in daily routines. Many people discover that meaningful change does not require overhauling everything at once but rather making steady, thoughtful adjustments. Replacing heavily processed snacks with fruit or nuts, adding fresh vegetables to each meal, or taking a moment before eating to pause and pray can shift the entire experience of nourishment. These steps seem small but gradually reshape how the body and spirit respond to food.

Integrating gratitude into meals deepens this transformation. In Scripture, mealtime prayers were not perfunctory but heartfelt acknowledgments of God's generosity. Practicing this posture helps reduce hurried eating and cultivates awareness of what is being consumed. Gratitude also counteracts the discontent that often drives unhealthy choices. When we give thanks, we see food less as a tool for coping or escape and more as a gift to be stewarded. This subtle shift has profound effects on both emotional and physical well-being.

Flexibility is another hallmark of a biblical meal framework. God's people ate according to what was available in their context, whether manna in the wilderness or fish by the Sea of Galilee. In the same way, applying biblical principles today is not about rigid meal plans but about adapting core values — whole foods, moderation, gratitude — to individual circumstances. A family in an urban apartment may have different options than someone with access to a garden, yet both can honor God through mindful choices.

Scientific insights help affirm these principles without becoming the primary focus. Research by Dr. David Katz (2014) shows that dietary patterns emphasizing whole foods and plant-based variety reduce inflammation, support heart health, and improve energy levels. These findings align closely with the foods highlighted in Scripture and provide reassurance that following God's wisdom is both spiritually meaningful and physically sound. When framed in this way, believers can feel confident that biblical guidance is not only relevant but also supported by modern understanding.

Community plays a vital role in sustaining these habits. Meals in the Bible were rarely solitary; they fostered connection, celebration, and shared responsibility. Eating together encourages accountability and strengthens relationships, while also providing opportunities to teach children gratitude and stewardship. Even occasional shared meals with friends or church groups can rekindle this sense of fellowship, transforming eating from an isolated act into a communal expression of faith.

Ultimately, practical biblical meal frameworks are about reorienting the heart. They invite us to slow down, to recognize God's provision, and to care for the body He entrusted to us. This is not about perfection but about progress — taking steps toward greater alignment with His design, one meal at a time. Over weeks and months, these small but intentional shifts accumulate into a lifestyle marked by balance, gratitude, and vitality. By embracing these principles, modern believers can reclaim eating as a sacred rhythm that nourishes both body and soul, reflecting God's goodness in every bite.

Part II. Biblical Practices for the Body

Foundations are essential, but understanding alone does not transform a life. The next step is practice — living out the principles of Scripture in tangible ways that shape how we eat, rest, and care for our bodies. The Bible is filled with rhythms that connect the physical and the spiritual. These are not empty rituals or cultural relics but timeless patterns designed by God to keep His people whole.

In this part of the book, we explore four central practices that directly involve the body: fasting, the use of sacred oils and remedies, water and purification, and Sabbath rest. Each of these disciplines addresses physical needs while nurturing deeper trust in God. Fasting humbles the appetite and clears space for focus and prayer. Sacred oils and remedies remind us that creation itself holds resources for healing and worship. Water, so central to life and renewal, carries both symbolic and practical meaning throughout Scripture. And Sabbath rest, perhaps the most countercultural of all, invites us to step out of relentless striving and rediscover the gift of restoration.

These practices are not meant to burden but to liberate. They reintroduce rhythms that modern life has largely forgotten — pauses in the noise, moments of intentional care, reminders of God's presence in ordinary actions. They are adaptable to any season or circumstance, whether life feels busy, uncertain, or calm. More importantly, they are invitations rather than obligations. The heart behind them matters more than the form they take.

As you read through these chapters, approach them not as a checklist but as opportunities to experiment with new ways of aligning body and spirit. Some practices may feel immediately life-giving; others may require patience and prayer to integrate fully. Each, however, offers a pathway back to harmony — a way of reclaiming the body as a vessel of worship and a participant in God's ongoing work of restoration.

Chapter 3: The Power of Fasting

Fasting in the Old and New Testament: Purposes and Patterns

Fasting is one of the most significant spiritual disciplines found throughout Scripture. It appears in both the Old and New Testaments, practiced by prophets, kings, and ordinary believers as a way to draw near to God, seek His guidance, and prepare for moments of great importance. While today fasting is often discussed in health and wellness circles for its physical benefits, the biblical understanding is far deeper. It is first and foremost an act of humility and dependence, a way of acknowledging that life's true sustenance comes from God rather than food alone.

In the Old Testament, fasting frequently accompanied repentance or times of seeking God's mercy. The nation of Israel fasted collectively during crises, such as in the book of Joel, where the people were called to humble themselves and cry out for God's deliverance. Individuals also fasted in personal lament or petition. David fasted when pleading for the life of his sick child. Ezra proclaimed a fast before leading the exiles back to Jerusalem, seeking God's protection on their journey. These examples reveal that fasting was not merely ritualistic but deeply relational, a physical posture that expressed the heart's longing for God's intervention and favor.

The prophets also challenged empty fasting. In Isaiah 58, God confronts those who fast outwardly but neglect justice, mercy, and compassion. The passage makes it clear that fasting without transformed behavior misses its purpose. True fasting, according to God, involves loosening the bonds of oppression, sharing food with the hungry, and caring for the vulnerable. This prophetic correction reminds us that fasting is never an end in itself but a means of aligning the heart with God's will.

In the New Testament, fasting continues to hold significance but is reframed through the life and teachings of Jesus. He Himself fasted for forty days in the wilderness, preparing for His public ministry and demonstrating complete dependence on the Father. His words in Matthew 6 assume that His followers will fast, saying "when you fast" rather than "if you fast," while warning against doing so to gain human approval. For Jesus, fasting is a private act of devotion, rooted in sincerity rather than performance.

The early church also practiced fasting regularly. Acts 13 records believers fasting and praying before sending Paul and Barnabas on their missionary journey. In Acts 14, fasting accompanies the appointment of new church leaders. These moments highlight how fasting was woven into decision-making and discernment, creating space for the Holy Spirit's guidance. Far from being an outdated practice, fasting remained central to the life of the early Christian community.

The patterns that emerge from these biblical accounts reveal several consistent purposes: seeking God in times of need, expressing repentance, preparing for significant callings, and cultivating deeper intimacy with Him. Fasting serves as a reset, breaking the cycle of constant consumption and reminding believers that their ultimate dependence is on God. It quiets distractions and sharpens spiritual awareness, often leading to clarity and renewed strength for the tasks ahead.

Fasting also carries an element of spiritual preparation. Throughout Scripture, significant encounters with God are often preceded by a period of abstaining from food. Moses fasted forty days before receiving the Ten Commandments. Esther called her people to fast before approaching the king to plead for their lives. These moments reveal fasting as a way of consecration — setting oneself apart to seek God's presence and strength for pivotal moments. This principle remains relevant today, not only for major life decisions but also for any situation that requires clarity and focus beyond what ordinary routines can provide.

An equally important aspect of fasting is its connection to prayer. The two are rarely separated in the biblical record. Fasting without prayer risks becoming a hollow exercise in willpower rather than a transformative spiritual discipline. When the body is denied its usual sustenance, the resulting hunger serves as a reminder to turn attention toward God. This redirection transforms physical longing into spiritual pursuit, creating space for deeper intimacy and dependence.

Modern applications of fasting can draw from these patterns while adapting to current circumstances. Believers today are not bound to replicate every detail of ancient practices but can embrace the underlying principles. Shorter fasts, partial fasts, or even abstaining from specific types of food can carry the same heart posture when approached with sincerity. The key is not the length or intensity of the fast but the humility and focus it cultivates. A single meal skipped in prayerful devotion may be more transformative than a lengthy fast undertaken for the wrong reasons.

Scientific research affirms many of the physical benefits of fasting while underscoring the wisdom of approaching it carefully. Studies by Dr. Valter Longo (2017) have highlighted how intermittent fasting supports cellular repair, reduces inflammation, and improves metabolic health. While these findings are valuable, they should never overshadow the spiritual purpose that makes biblical fasting unique. The health benefits are a gift, but the deeper reward is the closeness to God that fasting fosters.

Practicing fasting in community can also be deeply impactful. The Bible records several corporate fasts where entire groups humbled themselves together before God. This shared experience fosters unity and reminds believers that seeking God is not a solitary pursuit but one that strengthens the body of Christ as a whole. In today's context, church groups, families, or close friends may choose to fast together for guidance, healing, or intercession, encouraging one another throughout the process.

Ultimately, fasting is less about what is given up and more about what is gained. It creates space for realignment, helping believers quiet the noise of daily life and hear God's voice with greater clarity. It deepens dependence on Him and cultivates a humility that opens the door to transformation. Approached with the right heart, fasting remains as powerful today as it was in the days of the prophets and apostles, offering a way to step closer to the God who satisfies far beyond what food ever could.

Spiritual and Physical Benefits of Biblical Fasting

Fasting, when approached from a biblical perspective, brings together the spiritual and physical dimensions of life in a unique way. It is not only about abstaining from food but about entering a deeper space of dependence on God, quieting distractions, and allowing both the body and soul to reset. When practiced with the right heart, fasting becomes a pathway to clarity, renewal, and transformation that affects every part of life.

The spiritual benefits of fasting are woven throughout Scripture. One of the most profound is the way fasting heightens sensitivity to God's voice. When the usual rhythms of eating are interrupted, time and energy that would normally be devoted to meals can be redirected toward prayer and reflection. This shift creates room for deeper intimacy with God, allowing believers to hear Him more clearly and discern His guidance in areas of uncertainty. Moments of clarity often emerge not because God suddenly speaks louder but because fasting quiets the competing noise of daily life.

Fasting also serves as a powerful act of humility. In Scripture, humbling oneself before God often involved fasting, as seen in the examples of Ezra, Nehemiah, and the people of Nineveh. By willingly setting aside physical comfort, believers express a tangible recognition of their dependence on Him. This posture of humility opens the heart to repentance, gratitude, and deeper trust. It creates an inner space where transformation can take root, softening attitudes that may have been hardened by pride or distraction.

Another spiritual dimension of fasting is its role in intercession. Throughout the Bible, individuals and communities fasted when seeking God's intervention on behalf of others. Esther fasted before approaching the king to plead for her people's lives. The early church fasted before commissioning missionaries. In both cases, fasting was a way of seeking God's will with greater focus and urgency. This practice continues to be relevant today, offering believers a way to carry the burdens of loved ones or communities before God with renewed intentionality.

The physical benefits of fasting, while secondary to the spiritual purpose, are also significant. Modern research has uncovered insights that affirm what many biblical practices imply: periods of abstaining from food allow the body to repair and recalibrate in ways that constant eating does not. Intermittent fasting, for example, has been linked to improved insulin sensitivity, reduced inflammation, and enhanced cellular repair processes. These effects are not magical but reflect the body's God-designed ability to heal and renew itself when given time to rest from constant digestion.

Studies by Dr. Yoshinori Ohsumi, awarded the Nobel Prize in 2016, highlight the process of autophagy — the body's way of cleaning out damaged cells and regenerating healthier ones. This biological function is activated during fasting and illustrates a fascinating harmony between ancient spiritual disciplines and modern scientific understanding. While these findings should never overshadow fasting's primary spiritual purpose, they offer an encouraging reminder that God's design for the human body integrates physical and spiritual well-being in remarkable ways.

These physical benefits can also create a positive ripple effect in other areas of life. Improved energy, mental clarity, and reduced inflammation often support better focus during prayer, work, and relationships. While fasting is not undertaken for the sake of these outcomes, they serve as affirmations of how closely spiritual obedience and physical well-being are connected. This reinforces the biblical truth that body and soul are not separate compartments but part of an integrated whole designed to work in harmony.

Embracing fasting as both spiritual and physical renewal requires careful attention to the heart's posture. The purpose is not self-punishment or an attempt to earn favor from God but an act of love and trust. A fast undertaken out of pride or desire for recognition loses its power and can even become spiritually harmful. Jesus' teaching in Matthew 6 warns against fasting for public approval, calling instead for quiet devotion known only to the Father. This secrecy fosters authenticity and allows the focus to remain where it belongs — on God's presence and guidance.

Practical wisdom is also vital when incorporating fasting into modern life. Scripture portrays fasting as flexible, with variations ranging from complete abstinence to partial fasts like Daniel's choice of simple foods. This flexibility remains important today, particularly for individuals with health conditions, demanding schedules, or unique physical needs. A thoughtful approach respects the body's limits while still honoring the spiritual purpose behind the practice. Consulting medical guidance when needed is not a lack of faith but a recognition that stewardship includes caring wisely for the body.

Fasting also provides a unique training ground for self-control. By practicing restraint in one of life's most basic areas — food — believers strengthen the capacity to choose discipline over impulse in other areas, such as speech, finances, and relationships. This growth in self-control is not about rigid willpower but about yielding to the Spirit's work, learning to depend on God in moments of weakness rather than giving in to immediate cravings or distractions.

The transformative power of fasting becomes most evident over time. Many people describe an increased sensitivity to God's leading, a renewed sense of peace, and a release from anxieties they previously carried. These outcomes are not guaranteed, but they often emerge as byproducts of drawing near to God with an undivided heart. Physical health improvements may also become noticeable, from improved digestion to clearer thinking, further affirming the harmony of God's design.

Ultimately, the greatest benefit of biblical fasting is intimacy with God. Every hunger pang becomes an invitation to turn to Him in prayer. Every moment of weakness becomes an opportunity to experience His strength. Over days or weeks, fasting fosters a rhythm of seeking Him first, realigning priorities and reminding believers that He is the source of life itself. In this way, fasting is far more than abstaining from food; it is feasting on the presence of God, discovering in practice what Jesus meant when He said, "Man shall not live on bread alone, but on every word that comes from the mouth of God."

How to Fast Safely and Meaningfully in Modern Life

Fasting in the biblical sense was a deeply spiritual act, yet it unfolded in a context very different from today. Ancient diets were simpler, daily activity patterns were slower, and community life naturally supported rhythms of rest and prayer. Modern life, with its constant access to food, high-stress schedules, and complex health concerns, requires careful consideration when applying this practice. Fasting can still be profoundly meaningful, but doing it safely and intentionally ensures that it nurtures both body and spirit rather than causing harm or frustration.

The first step is clarifying purpose. In Scripture, fasting was never random; it was always tied to seeking God, humbling oneself, or preparing for something significant. Before beginning, ask what you are seeking through this time of fasting. Is it greater clarity in decision-making? Deeper intimacy with God? A heart reset from distraction or complacency? Setting a clear spiritual intention transforms fasting from a physical challenge into an act of worship. Without this focus, it risks becoming little more than skipped meals.

Equally important is understanding your physical readiness. While biblical fasting ranges from partial to complete abstention, modern application must take into account individual health conditions, work demands, and energy levels. Those with medical concerns such as diabetes, low blood pressure, or eating disorders should consult a qualified health professional before attempting any fast. Stewardship of the body includes acknowledging its limitations. In some cases, modifying the fast — for example, abstaining from specific foods rather than all food — may be the wisest approach while still honoring the spiritual principle behind it.

Preparing for a fast is just as vital as the fast itself. Suddenly stopping food intake can shock the body, leading to headaches, irritability, and fatigue. Gradually reducing processed foods, caffeine, and heavy meals in the days leading up to a fast eases the transition and helps maintain focus on the spiritual purpose rather than physical discomfort. Planning prayer times, setting aside quiet moments, and informing close family or friends of your intentions can also reduce unnecessary stress and provide support throughout the process.

Choosing the right type of fast depends on personal circumstances and discernment. Full fasts, where only water is consumed, can be powerful but are best kept short and approached cautiously. Partial fasts, such as Daniel's choice to eat only vegetables and water, may be more sustainable for longer periods while still cultivating humility and focus. Some believers choose to fast from specific meals, like breakfast or dinner, creating windows for prayer and reflection without compromising health. The key is aligning the form of the fast with both spiritual goals and practical realities, ensuring it deepens devotion rather than becoming an unmanageable burden.

Breaking the fast well is as significant as beginning it. After any period of abstaining, the body is more sensitive to what is reintroduced. Starting with light, nourishing foods such as fruits, vegetables, and broths helps avoid discomfort and supports the body's natural rhythms. This gradual approach mirrors the spirit of fasting itself — measured, mindful, and rooted in stewardship rather than excess. Ending with gratitude, taking a moment to reflect on what God revealed during the fast, transforms the conclusion into an act of worship rather than simply a return to routine.

Sustaining the spiritual gains from a fast often depends on what follows. Many people experience clarity and renewed intimacy with God during fasting, only to return quickly to old habits. Carrying forward the lessons learned — whether a deeper prayer life, greater dependence on Scripture, or heightened awareness of God's provision — ensures the fast becomes a foundation rather than an isolated event. This may involve setting aside regular times for prayer or choosing periodic mini-fasts to stay aligned with the rhythms God has cultivated during the longer fast.

Fasting can also extend beyond food to other areas where distraction or overindulgence dulls spiritual sensitivity. Some may fast from digital media, unnecessary spending, or constant noise to create space for God's voice. While these are not replacements for traditional fasting, they share the principle of surrender — intentionally laying something down to focus on what matters most. Combining a food fast with another form of abstention can be particularly powerful, especially in a culture saturated with constant stimulation.

It is essential to approach fasting with humility rather than comparison. The purpose is not to outdo others in duration or strictness but to pursue personal transformation. Jesus' teaching to keep fasting private underscores this principle. The value lies in authenticity, not appearance. Whether the fast lasts a day or a week, whether it is full or partial, what matters is the posture of the heart and the willingness to respond to God's leading.

Modern research continues to affirm the health benefits of fasting, but for believers, these outcomes remain secondary. The true reward is the alignment of body and spirit with God's purposes. Each pang of hunger can serve as a reminder to pray, each moment of weakness an opportunity to rely on His strength. In this way, fasting becomes less about deprivation and more about exchange — trading self-reliance for dependence on God, anxiety for peace, distraction for clarity.

Practiced thoughtfully, fasting can become a steady rhythm rather than a rare event. It provides a means of recalibrating life when stress accumulates, decisions loom, or spiritual dryness sets in. It creates a sacred pause in a world that rarely stops, inviting believers to step out of routine and listen. In doing so, fasting remains one of the most powerful ways to bridge the ancient and modern — a discipline as relevant today as it was in the days of prophets and apostles, capable of renewing both the inner and outer life in profound ways.

Chapter 4: Sacred Oils and Biblical Remedies

Frankincense, Myrrh, and Olive Oil: Scriptural Uses and Symbolism

Throughout the pages of Scripture, certain natural substances stand out for their profound spiritual and practical significance. Frankincense, myrrh, and olive oil are among the most notable, appearing in both Old and New Testament narratives. These elements were not merely commodities; they held deep symbolic meaning, played central roles in worship, and were often associated with healing, consecration, and divine presence. Understanding their role in biblical times helps us appreciate why they continue to captivate believers today and what lessons they offer for modern spiritual practice.

Frankincense, a resin obtained from the Boswellia tree, was one of the key ingredients in the sacred incense used in temple worship. Exodus 30 describes a specific blend of spices — including frankincense — burned before the Ark of the Covenant as an offering to God. The rising smoke symbolized the prayers of the people ascending to heaven, a theme echoed in Psalm 141:2 and later in Revelation 5:8. This association between frankincense and prayer conveys an enduring truth: the fragrance of devotion is pleasing to God, and the act of lifting hearts toward Him carries profound spiritual weight.

Myrrh, another resin, was used for both sacred and practical purposes. In the Old Testament, it appeared in anointing oils and perfumes, symbolizing holiness and consecration. Myrrh was also valued for its preservative properties, which explains its presence at Jesus' burial (John 19:39) and why it was offered to Him mixed with wine during His crucifixion (Mark 15:23). This dual use — both sacred and somber — reflects myrrh's role in moments of deep significance, from worship to mourning, and highlights how biblical healing and worship practices were deeply integrated into daily life.

Olive oil held an even broader role in Scripture, permeating almost every aspect of ancient life. It was used for cooking, lighting lamps, anointing kings and priests, and even in healing rituals. James 5:14 instructs believers to anoint the sick with oil in prayer, a practice rooted in the belief that physical and spiritual restoration are intertwined. Olive oil symbolized abundance, blessing, and the presence of the Holy Spirit, seen most vividly in the anointing of David in 1 Samuel 16. Its widespread use in biblical times made it both a practical necessity and a profound spiritual emblem.

These substances also carried prophetic weight. The gifts of gold, frankincense, and myrrh brought by the Magi to the infant Jesus (Matthew 2:11) were not random tokens of wealth but carefully chosen symbols: gold for kingship, frankincense for divinity, and myrrh for suffering and sacrifice. This moment encapsulated the fullness of Christ's identity and mission, showing how natural elements could convey profound theological truths.

The frequent mention of these materials underscores the biblical pattern of using tangible, earthly substances to point toward spiritual realities. They bridged the physical and the divine, reminding God's people that His presence permeated all of life — from worship in the temple to the healing of wounds. Exploring these elements helps modern readers see that biblical faith has always been embodied, calling believers to honor God not only with words and thoughts but also through physical expressions of devotion and care.

The symbolism of these elements is further deepened by the way they are woven into covenantal moments. Olive oil anointed prophets, priests, and kings, setting them apart for sacred service. This act of anointing was more than ceremonial; it represented the Spirit of God equipping individuals for their calling. David's anointing by Samuel signaled God's choice and favor, a moment later affirmed by the Spirit's power resting upon him. The fragrance of frankincense in the temple and the bittersweet presence of myrrh in burial rites remind us that God's story encompasses both joy and sorrow, victory and sacrifice.

Understanding the cultural and symbolic weight of these substances also reframes their use in modern contexts. While some today may incorporate oils or incense into personal prayer, the deeper lesson is about intentionality. The biblical pattern was never about superstition or empty ritual but about setting ordinary things apart for holy purposes. A simple act, like lighting a lamp or anointing with oil, became a reminder of God's presence because it was done in faith and reverence. Reclaiming this posture allows believers today to integrate sacred meaning into everyday life without reducing these practices to trends or novelty.

Modern research into these natural substances has uncovered properties that, while secondary to their spiritual meaning, affirm their value. Frankincense has been studied for its potential anti-inflammatory effects, and myrrh for its antimicrobial qualities. Olive oil, central to the Mediterranean diet, is recognized for its heart-protective benefits and richness in antioxidants. While these findings should never overshadow their symbolic role, they illustrate the harmony between God's creation and human well-being. What was once used in worship also provided tangible benefits for the body, demonstrating how divine wisdom permeates even practical aspects of life.

Equally important is remembering that the true power never resided in the substances themselves. Scripture consistently points beyond the symbol to the God who gave it meaning. Anointing oil was not magical; its effectiveness depended on faith and obedience. Incense did not guarantee answered prayers; it represented hearts genuinely turned toward God. This distinction safeguards against treating these elements as talismans and keeps focus on the relationship they are meant to foster. For modern believers, the enduring lesson of frankincense, myrrh, and olive oil is to live with greater awareness of God's presence in the physical world. Meals can become acts of gratitude, simple rituals can become reminders of holiness, and the care of the body can reflect reverence for the Creator. When ordinary things are dedicated to God, they are transformed, not because their substance changes but because their meaning does. This integration of faith and daily life echoes the biblical vision of worship that is holistic, embodied, and ever mindful of the sacred in the ordinary.

The Healing Role of Herbs and Anointing Practices

The Bible's portrayal of healing is deeply holistic, uniting body, mind, and spirit in a way that modern culture often separates. Among its many practices, the use of herbs and anointing oils stands out as a bridge between the physical and spiritual. These natural elements were not merely medicinal; they carried symbolic meaning and were frequently employed as part of prayer and worship. Understanding how they were used in Scripture offers valuable insight into God's design for caring for the body and integrating faith into daily life.

Herbs appear throughout the biblical narrative, often as part of both food and healing practices. In Genesis, plants and seeds are described as gifts for nourishment, and this provision extends naturally to their restorative qualities. Spices and herbs such as hyssop, aloe, and balm of Gilead were well known in the ancient Near East for their soothing and purifying properties. Hyssop, for instance, was used in ceremonial cleansing rituals (Psalm 51:7) and also functioned as a disinfectant in practical contexts. This dual purpose reflects the biblical pattern of blending physical care with spiritual symbolism.

Olive oil, while central to cooking and worship, also played a key role in healing. The parable of the Good Samaritan describes the wounded man being treated with oil and wine, a combination used both to cleanse and soothe injuries. This simple act of mercy illustrates how everyday substances were applied in compassionate care, reminding believers that healing often begins with attentiveness and practical love. In James 5:14, the call to anoint the sick with oil and pray over them reinforces this link between tangible action and divine intervention, showing that physical touch and faith-filled prayer were never meant to be separated.

Anointing in biblical times went beyond physical application; it marked moments of consecration and blessing. Priests, prophets, and kings were set apart through the pouring of oil, symbolizing the presence and empowerment of the Holy Spirit. When this practice intersected with healing, it pointed to the reality that restoration is not just about repairing the body but about bringing the whole person into alignment with God's purposes. The anointing of the sick, therefore, was as much about invoking God's presence as it was about addressing physical symptoms. The medicinal qualities of herbs and oils used in biblical times align strikingly with modern scientific findings. For example, myrrh and frankincense — both common in ancient anointing blends — have been studied for their antimicrobial and anti-inflammatory properties. Olive oil is known for its healthy fats and antioxidants, which support heart health and reduce inflammation. While these benefits should never be exaggerated or treated as miraculous cures, they demonstrate the harmony between God's creation and human well-being. Biblical practices often anticipated principles that modern science is only now beginning to understand.

These insights remind us that the value of herbs and anointing oils lies not in superstition but in stewardship. God provided resources in creation to nurture and sustain life, inviting His people to use them wisely. When incorporated with prayer, gratitude, and humility, these practices become opportunities to acknowledge God as the ultimate healer. They invite believers to see the natural world not as separate from spiritual life but as a canvas through which God's care and provision are revealed.

This integration of physical remedies with prayerful intention also teaches something about the character of biblical healing. The focus was rarely on quick fixes or isolated symptoms but on restoring wholeness. In the prophetic writings, God's promise to heal His people often included spiritual renewal and communal restoration. Using herbs and oils in prayer mirrored this holistic vision. They were signs of care for the body while simultaneously pointing hearts back to the Giver of life.

Practical application today draws on these same principles rather than rigidly copying ancient methods. A believer might use olive oil in prayer over someone who is ill, not because the oil itself holds mystical power, but because it symbolizes consecration and invites God's presence into the moment. Similarly, incorporating natural foods and herbs into meals can become an act of gratitude and stewardship, acknowledging God's provision rather than chasing the latest wellness trend. This approach guards against two extremes — neglecting the physical entirely or overemphasizing it in search of miracle cures.

The communal aspect of these practices is equally significant. James 5:14 places anointing within the context of church community, where elders pray for the sick together. Healing, in the biblical view, was rarely a solitary pursuit. It was something sought and celebrated within the body of believers, reinforcing bonds of compassion and mutual care. In a modern culture often characterized by isolation, reclaiming this collective dimension can be deeply restorative. Inviting trusted friends or church leaders into moments of prayer and anointing fosters accountability and reminds individuals that they are not alone in their struggles.

Scientific understanding, while secondary to faith, enriches this conversation by affirming the wisdom embedded in these practices. Studies have explored how aromatic compounds in herbs like frankincense may influence emotional calm, while olive oil's nutrient profile supports cardiovascular health. Even simple acts of touch, like anointing someone during prayer, have been shown to reduce stress and foster connection. These findings do not diminish the spiritual dimension but instead highlight how God's creation is intricately designed to support both body and soul.

The enduring lesson is that healing in Scripture was never about separating the sacred from the ordinary. Herbs, oils, and anointing practices reminded God's people that every aspect of life — what they ate, how they cared for wounds, how they prayed — could be an expression of worship. Bringing these principles into modern life invites believers to approach health with reverence rather than fear, recognizing that God's provision often comes through both prayer and practical means.

Ultimately, the healing role of herbs and anointing practices points beyond the elements themselves to the One who heals. The olive oil, the fragrant resins, and the cleansing herbs were conduits for faith, not substitutes for it. Their use called people to remember that true restoration flows from God's presence and promises. By blending prayer, humility, and wise use of creation's gifts, believers today can honor this biblical vision of healing — one that integrates body and spirit in a way that remains profoundly relevant in the modern world.

How to Incorporate Oils Ethically and Practically Today

The use of oils in Scripture carries deep symbolic and practical meaning, but applying these practices today requires both discernment and humility. Modern interest in essential oils and natural remedies has grown significantly, yet this popularity sometimes leads to confusion or misuse. Some view oils as miracle cures, while others dismiss them as irrelevant to faith. A balanced biblical perspective offers a different path — one that honors the original intent of these practices while applying them responsibly in a contemporary setting.

The first consideration is purpose. In the Bible, oils were used for anointing, consecration, and healing, always pointing back to God's presence rather than to the substance itself. This principle remains vital today. Using olive oil or frankincense in prayer can serve as a meaningful reminder of God's nearness, but it should never be treated as a shortcut to spiritual power or a guarantee of physical results. The ethical use of oils begins with this posture of humility, recognizing them as tools to aid devotion rather than ends in themselves.

Practical application also requires understanding the limits of oils. While many possess beneficial properties, they are not replacements for medical care or treatment for serious conditions. James 5:14 places anointing with oil alongside prayer, not in place of wise action or professional help. Ethical practice means using oils as part of a holistic approach — combining prayer, healthy living, and appropriate medical attention when needed. This perspective helps avoid extremes, whether over-reliance on oils or neglect of their potential value.

Sourcing and quality are additional factors to consider. In biblical times, oils were pressed or distilled from plants and resins in their purest form. Today's commercial market varies widely in purity and ethical standards. Choosing oils that are responsibly sourced, free of harmful additives, and transparently labeled honors both the body and the integrity of God's creation. It also reflects the biblical principle of stewardship, ensuring that what we use in worship or care does not exploit people or the environment.

When incorporating oils into spiritual practice, simplicity often carries the most meaning. A small amount of olive oil used in personal or communal prayer can be profoundly symbolic without needing elaborate rituals. Likewise, diffusing frankincense during a time of reflection or applying oil gently during intercessory prayer can create a tangible reminder of God's presence. The act itself should draw attention to Him, not to the oil or the person performing the anointing.

Using oils in daily life can also become an act of mindfulness that strengthens spiritual awareness. A simple prayer of thanksgiving when preparing food with olive oil, or pausing to reflect on God's provision when lighting a lamp-scented candle, turns ordinary routines into moments of worship. This approach keeps faith grounded in everyday life, reminding believers that sacredness is not confined to church walls but extends into kitchens, homes, and workplaces.

Community use of oils continues to hold significance as well. In Scripture, anointing was often public, performed by leaders or elders as part of prayer for healing or commissioning. Practicing this today can foster deeper connection within church communities. When anointing someone who is ill or burdened, the focus shifts away from individual striving and toward collective support and intercession. These moments also reaffirm that the body of Christ carries one another's burdens, transforming care into a shared spiritual experience rather than an isolated act.

Awareness of cultural sensitivity is also important. Oils and incense have spiritual significance in many faith traditions outside Christianity. When incorporating them into prayer or worship, clarity of intent matters. The aim is not to adopt foreign practices uncritically but to reclaim a biblical understanding that is rooted in Scripture. Explaining the symbolism — such as olive oil representing consecration or frankincense reflecting prayer rising to God — helps prevent misunderstanding and ensures the focus remains on honoring Him.

The ethical dimension extends to how oils are spoken about and shared. In a culture saturated with marketing claims, it is easy to blur the line between faith and commerce. Overstating what oils can do, especially in the context of healing, risks misleading others and undermines the credibility of genuine spiritual practices. A Christ-centered approach avoids exaggeration and invites others to experience the deeper meaning without pressure or unrealistic promises.

Practical steps for incorporating oils might include setting aside a small vial of olive oil for personal prayer or church use, choosing moments of significance such as praying over someone entering a new season of life or seeking comfort during illness. Oils can also be incorporated into corporate worship on special occasions, such as commissioning leaders or during times of communal repentance and renewal. These practices, kept simple and grounded in humility, remind participants of God's presence in a tangible yet unobtrusive way.

Ultimately, ethical and practical use of oils today is about balance — embracing their symbolic richness and natural benefits without allowing them to overshadow the One they point toward. They are part of creation, designed to serve and bless rather than dominate attention. When used thoughtfully, they become tools that elevate prayer, mark sacred moments, and encourage gratitude. This approach invites believers to recover the depth of biblical traditions while engaging modern life with discernment, ensuring that every act of anointing, every fragrance rising in prayer, directs hearts back to God as the true source of healing and restoration.

Chapter 5: Water, Purification, and Renewal

Living Water: Symbolism and Physical Importance

Water flows through the entire biblical narrative, carrying both practical and profound spiritual meaning. It is central to life itself, sustaining the body and nourishing creation, yet it is also a recurring symbol of cleansing, renewal, and divine provision. When Scripture speaks of "living water," it refers not only to streams and springs but to the life-giving presence of God Himself. Understanding this dual meaning deepens the way we view both physical hydration and the spiritual refreshment God offers.

In the physical sense, water was essential in the daily lives of biblical communities. Located in arid regions, access to clean water determined survival. Wells and springs became central gathering points for families and travelers. The significance of water in daily routines — from washing hands to preparing food — made it a natural symbol of purity and refreshment. This context illuminates why many of Jesus' teachings about water, such as His conversation with the Samaritan woman in John 4, carried such immediate resonance for His listeners. When He promised living water that would quench thirst forever, He spoke into a reality where water scarcity was a constant concern.

Water's role in ritual purification also runs deep in the Old Testament. Ceremonial washings were prescribed for priests before entering the tabernacle, and the people were often called to cleanse themselves as an outward sign of inner repentance. The use of water in these rituals pointed beyond hygiene to a deeper truth: God's holiness invites His people into purity, and cleansing symbolizes the renewal He offers. The prophet Ezekiel spoke of God sprinkling clean water on His people to cleanse them from impurities (Ezekiel 36:25), a promise later echoed in the New Testament's language of baptism.

Baptism itself becomes the most vivid expression of water's spiritual symbolism. When John baptized in the Jordan River, and later when Jesus commanded His disciples to baptize in the name of the Father,

Son, and Holy Spirit, the act represented death to the old life and rebirth into the new. This imagery builds on the Old Testament's themes of water as both cleansing and life-giving. The crossing of the Red Sea and later the Jordan River into the Promised Land also foreshadowed this idea — moments when water marked the threshold into a new covenant reality.

The metaphor of living water reaches its fullest meaning in Jesus Himself. He not only offers water that quenches thirst but declares in John 7 that rivers of living water will flow from within those who believe in Him, referring to the Holy Spirit. This is a shift from external cleansing to internal renewal. The imagery moves from washing the body to transforming the heart, a promise of ongoing refreshment and vitality that flows from God's presence within.

From a physical perspective, modern understanding underscores water's indispensable role in health. Proper hydration supports every system in the body, from regulating temperature and aiding digestion to maintaining cognitive clarity and joint health. Chronic dehydration, often overlooked, can contribute to fatigue, headaches, and diminished focus. This physical reality reinforces why biblical imagery of water as life-giving resonates so deeply; the body's dependence on water mirrors the soul's dependence on God.

The parallels between physical and spiritual thirst invite a deeper reflection on what truly satisfies. Just as the body signals dehydration with fatigue or dizziness, the soul signals spiritual dryness through restlessness, anxiety, or disconnection. Many attempt to quench this deeper thirst through distraction or achievement, yet the longing remains. Scripture's promise of living water addresses this very need, offering a source of renewal that cannot be found in external circumstances. This imagery speaks to the core human experience: the search for something enduring in a world where everything else runs dry. Water's presence in key biblical narratives also highlights God's faithfulness in providing for His people. In the wilderness, God brought water from a rock to sustain Israel when they faced thirst. In Revelation, the final vision of the new heaven and earth includes a river of the water of life, clear as crystal, flowing from the throne of God. These bookends of Scripture — from provision in the desert to abundance in eternity — reveal water as a consistent sign of God's care. It sustains not only life but hope, reminding believers that their journey is held in His hands.

In daily life, integrating this symbolism can deepen both faith and practical health. Choosing to drink water with mindfulness, offering a prayer of thanks, or reflecting on Jesus' promise of living water during moments of weariness can transform an ordinary act into spiritual nourishment. The physical act of hydrating becomes a reminder of the Spirit's presence, turning a basic need into an opportunity for connection with God. Such practices anchor faith in routine, allowing spiritual truths to permeate the simplest moments.

Scientific insights further affirm why water carries such profound meaning. Research consistently shows that even mild dehydration affects mood, focus, and energy levels. Athletes and medical professionals alike emphasize hydration as foundational for recovery and resilience. These findings align seamlessly with the biblical portrayal of water as essential for renewal. While Scripture does not speak in scientific terms, its consistent imagery anticipates truths modern research continues to validate — that water is life-giving on every level.

Ultimately, living water points beyond physical sustenance to the deeper reality of God's presence. It invites believers to receive what only He can give: a source of refreshment that does not run dry. This promise does not remove life's challenges but provides strength within them, offering peace that persists even in seasons of drought. To drink of this living water is to enter into ongoing communion with God, where renewal flows not just once but continually, shaping every part of life.

Ritual Cleansing in Scripture and Its Modern Meaning

Ritual cleansing is one of the oldest and most enduring practices in the biblical narrative. It appears in laws, ceremonies, and symbolic acts throughout both the Old and New Testaments, pointing to humanity's need for purity before approaching God. While modern readers may be tempted to view these practices as purely cultural or outdated, their underlying meaning continues to offer profound insight into spiritual life and personal renewal today.

In the Old Testament, cleansing rituals were woven into the fabric of Israel's covenant life. The book of Leviticus outlines detailed instructions for washing after contact with unclean things, for purification following childbirth, and for priests preparing to serve in the tabernacle. These acts were not simply about physical hygiene, though they undoubtedly promoted health in a pre-modern world. They served a symbolic purpose: to remind God's people of His holiness and their need for purification to enter His presence. The very process of washing with water — tangible, repeated, and visible — impressed upon them the reality of God's call to be set apart.

One of the most striking examples is the priestly preparation before entering the holy place. Before offering sacrifices or handling sacred objects, priests were required to wash their hands and feet at the bronze basin (Exodus 30:17-21). This was more than routine; it signified readiness and reverence. By cleansing themselves, the priests acknowledged that service before God required both physical and spiritual preparation. The washing did not make them righteous, but it symbolized the posture of heart and body necessary to approach the Holy One.

Cleansing rituals were also connected to moments of repentance and renewal. The psalmist's plea in Psalm 51, "Wash me, and I will be whiter than snow," uses physical imagery to express a longing for inner transformation. The prophets often echoed this theme, calling Israel to wash themselves and turn from sin as a sign of returning to God. Here, the act of cleansing became a metaphor for spiritual restoration — not just removing dirt, but symbolizing a fresh start.

In the New Testament, these themes take on new depth. Baptism emerges as the ultimate cleansing ritual, representing both repentance and rebirth. John the Baptist's ministry centered on calling people to confess their sins and be baptized in the Jordan River, preparing the way for Christ. Jesus Himself was baptized, not because He needed cleansing, but to identify fully with humanity and to fulfill righteousness. Later, baptism became the defining act of initiation into the Christian community, symbolizing dying to the old self and rising into new life.

Beyond baptism, Jesus redefined purity itself. In His teaching, true defilement came not from external contact but from the condition of the heart (Mark 7:15). This shift did not abolish the symbolism of washing but deepened it. Cleansing was no longer about strict adherence to external regulations; it pointed toward the inner renewal made possible through Him. The ritual remained meaningful, but its ultimate fulfillment was found in the transformation of the heart by God's Spirit. This deeper understanding of cleansing shapes how believers can approach similar practices today. Water continues to symbolize renewal in Christian baptism, but it also serves as a reminder in everyday life. Acts as simple as washing hands, bathing, or even drinking water can become moments to reflect on God's continual work of cleansing and restoring. These reminders do not replace the significance of baptism or formal rituals, but they allow the truth behind them to permeate ordinary routines.

Modern faith practices inspired by biblical cleansing do not need to replicate ancient laws to carry meaning. A personal prayer before showering, a symbolic washing of hands before entering a time of prayer, or even setting aside a specific day for renewal can embody the same posture of humility and preparation seen in Scripture. The essence lies not in the outward act alone but in the heart's willingness to approach God with reverence and openness.

Scientific insights further enrich this conversation. Ritual washing, long before germ theory, carried tangible health benefits by preventing the spread of illness. Modern hygiene practices mirror this wisdom, showing how God's commands often protected His people in practical ways while also pointing to spiritual truths. This harmony between physical and spiritual realities invites believers to see God's care woven into creation, where obedience brings both symbolic and real-world blessings.

Community remains central to cleansing imagery as well. Baptism in the early church was a public declaration, a visible sign of joining the family of faith. Even today, communal rituals — whether baptisms, renewal services, or corporate prayers for cleansing — remind believers that spiritual growth is not solitary. Participating in these acts together fosters accountability and shared commitment, encouraging one another toward holiness and gratitude.

The ultimate meaning of cleansing points beyond water itself to the transformation made possible through Christ. His sacrifice fulfills what the rituals of the Old Covenant foreshadowed, offering a cleansing that reaches the heart and conscience. Hebrews 10:22 captures this beautifully: "Let us draw near to God with a sincere heart and with the full assurance that faith brings, having our hearts sprinkled to cleanse us from a guilty conscience and having our bodies washed with pure water." This verse unites inward and outward renewal, showing that the work God accomplishes in the heart is inseparable from how it is lived out in the body.

For modern believers, embracing this vision can be as simple as creating rhythms of intentional reflection. A day set aside for quiet prayer and confession, beginning with a symbolic washing, can serve as a reset in seasons of weariness or distraction. Parents can incorporate meaningful washing rituals into family life, teaching children about God's forgiveness and the fresh start He offers. Churches might integrate corporate prayers of cleansing during communion or special services, echoing the continuity between ancient practices and the grace now revealed in Christ.

Ultimately, ritual cleansing invites believers into a life of ongoing renewal. It reminds them that God's presence is holy, His mercy is abundant, and His invitation to draw near is always open. By reclaiming the heart behind these practices — humility, preparation, and gratitude — modern Christians can experience the profound symbolism of water in a way that shapes both their faith and daily lives.

Practical Ways to Integrate Water for Healing and Peace

Water is one of the simplest yet most profound gifts of creation. In Scripture, it symbolizes renewal and cleansing, but it also sustains life in the most tangible way. Integrating water intentionally into daily rhythms can bridge physical health and spiritual restoration, allowing believers to experience its benefits in a way that nurtures both body and soul. This approach does not require elaborate rituals; rather, it invites a deeper awareness of God's presence through everyday practices.

One of the most immediate ways water contributes to well-being is through hydration. While this seems basic, dehydration is surprisingly common and often contributes to fatigue, headaches, and irritability. Regularly drinking water supports mental clarity, energy, and overall resilience. Turning this simple act into a moment of gratitude can transform it from a routine habit into an opportunity for worship. Pausing to thank God for His provision with each glass reframes hydration as a reminder of the living water Christ offers to the soul.

Bathing or immersion can also serve as a powerful tool for renewal. In biblical times, washing the body symbolized preparation for prayer, worship, or sacred service. Modern life rarely carries this same sense of reverence, yet intentionally reclaiming it can be transformative. A shower or bath, approached mindfully, becomes more than physical cleansing. It becomes an invitation to release stress, pray for renewal, and remember God's promises of washing away burdens. Some find value in combining this time with Scripture meditation, silently reflecting on passages about renewal or peace.

Spending time near natural water sources offers another layer of healing. Streams, lakes, and oceans evoke awe and quiet the mind, creating space for prayer and reflection. Many find that the sound of moving water fosters a sense of calm that encourages deeper connection with God. This aligns with Jesus' own example; He often withdrew to quiet places, and while not always near water, the principle of retreating into creation for renewal remains consistent. Choosing moments to walk by a riverbank or sit beside the sea can serve as a form of contemplative prayer, reconnecting body and spirit with the Creator.

Water can also become part of intentional rituals for transition or reset. Marking the beginning of a new season — whether a new year, a major life decision, or a personal commitment — with a symbolic washing can provide a tangible reminder of God's grace and fresh starts. This does not replace baptism but builds on its meaning, reinforcing the truth that renewal is ongoing. Even washing hands or face with prayerful intention can become a quiet act of consecration, especially in moments of stress or before entering important responsibilities.

Integrating water into spiritual practice also extends to how it is used in community. Shared rituals, such as group prayer accompanied by handwashing or symbolic pouring of water, can foster unity and remind participants of their collective dependence on God. In church settings, this might take the form of communal renewal services where water is used to signify new beginnings or reconciliation. These moments create shared memory and deepen the sense of belonging, reinforcing that healing and peace are not solitary pursuits but experienced together in the body of Christ.

Water's role in calming the nervous system is another reason it lends itself so naturally to practices of peace. The sound of flowing water, whether from a fountain, rain, or ocean waves, has been shown in modern studies to lower stress levels and slow the heart rate. Engaging with water through quiet observation — watching ripples on a pond or listening to rainfall — can create a meditative space that opens the heart to prayer. These moments of stillness invite reflection and can become anchors in seasons of uncertainty or transition.

Practical integration also involves acknowledging the gift of clean water and responding with gratitude and stewardship. Many in the world still lack access to safe drinking water, a reality that Scripture calls believers to address through compassion and action. Incorporating prayers for those in need, supporting clean water initiatives, or simply practicing mindful conservation connects personal renewal to a broader expression of love and justice. This perspective transforms even small acts, like limiting waste or sharing resources, into participation in God's work of restoration.

The beauty of water practices lies in their accessibility. No specialized tools or advanced knowledge are required. A simple glass of water, a quiet walk by a stream, or a few moments in the shower can become opportunities to reconnect with God's promises. The key is intentionality — approaching these moments with openness rather than rushing through them. Over time, these small acts form a rhythm that weaves peace and renewal into everyday life, gradually reshaping how we experience God's presence.

Ultimately, water in Scripture points beyond itself to the source of all healing and peace. Each sip, each cleansing, each quiet moment by a river invites believers to remember the living water offered by Christ. It is this water that satisfies the deepest thirst and sustains the soul through every season. By integrating water into daily rhythms with gratitude and reverence, modern believers can live out a timeless truth: that God's gifts in creation are meant to draw us back to Him, refreshing both body and spirit in ways that are as simple as they are profound.

Chapter 6: Rest and the Sabbath Principle

God's Rhythm of Work and Rest: Why It Matters for Health

From the opening chapters of Genesis, Scripture reveals a divine pattern woven into creation itself — six days of purposeful work followed by a day of rest. This rhythm was not only given to humanity but modeled by God Himself. After forming the heavens and the earth, He rested on the seventh day, blessing it and setting it apart as holy. This was not rest from exhaustion, for God does not grow weary, but rest that established a sacred pace for human life. Recognizing and aligning with this rhythm offers profound implications for physical health, emotional balance, and spiritual well-being.

The command to honor the Sabbath, later given to Israel in the Ten Commandments, was not merely a legalistic requirement but a gift. It served as a reminder that life is sustained by God's provision, not human striving. For an agricultural people whose survival depended on continual labor, ceasing from work required trust. It declared that even in rest, God remained faithful to provide. This principle remains just as relevant in modern culture, where productivity is often idolized and rest is undervalued. Choosing to pause affirms that worth is not defined by output but by relationship with the Creator.

Physically, rest is essential for health and longevity. Modern research confirms what Scripture has long implied: chronic overwork and lack of restorative rest lead to increased stress, hormonal imbalances, and heightened risk of disease. Studies on sleep and recovery consistently demonstrate that periods of intentional rest enhance immune function, improve mental clarity, and restore emotional resilience. This aligns with the biblical vision of rest not as laziness but as renewal — a necessary counterbalance to meaningful labor.

Emotionally, observing rhythms of rest cultivates peace and perspective. When life is lived in constant motion, anxiety and burnout easily take root. The Sabbath principle invites believers to step back, breathe, and remember who holds the world together. In doing so, it breaks the illusion of self-sufficiency and creates space for gratitude. The act of resting becomes worship, a declaration that God's presence is enough even when tasks remain unfinished.

Spiritually, rest serves as preparation. Ceasing from work is not an escape from purpose but a way of re-centering on it. The Gospels describe Jesus frequently withdrawing to solitary places for prayer, often after intense periods of ministry. These moments of retreat replenished Him for continued service and reflect a model for modern discipleship. Rest, rightly understood, is not disengagement from life but realignment with God's design for it.

Honoring God's rhythm of rest also nurtures relationships. Families that intentionally pause from constant activity often find space for meaningful connection that busy schedules crowd out. Meals become unhurried, conversations deepen, and shared worship becomes more central. This aligns with the biblical vision of the Sabbath as a communal celebration, not merely an individual retreat. In the Old Testament, the Sabbath was a day for families and communities to gather, rejoice, and remember God's deliverance. Reclaiming even part of this rhythm can transform modern households, fostering bonds that strengthen emotional and spiritual health.

There is also an element of humility in practicing rest. Taking a day to step back from work acknowledges human limits and affirms God's sovereignty. It resists the cultural pressure to find identity in busyness and productivity. This humility frees believers from the endless cycle of striving and comparison, reminding them that God values presence and faithfulness more than constant activity. In this way, rest becomes an act of trust — a quiet proclamation that God's care is sufficient.

Modern application of Sabbath principles does not always require strict adherence to a single day. While traditional observance centers on one day of rest each week, the heart of the command is to cultivate a rhythm that honors God and renews the body and mind. For some, this may involve setting aside Sunday for worship and family time. For others, particularly those in demanding schedules, it may mean carving out intentional spaces within the week for prayer, reflection, and rest. What matters is not legalism but alignment with the spirit of God's design.

Practical ways to honor this rhythm can include creating boundaries with work, turning off digital distractions, and approaching rest with purpose rather than passivity. A walk in nature, a quiet meal shared with loved ones, or time spent in Scripture and prayer can all serve as ways to enter into the gift of rest. These practices allow the soul to recalibrate and prepare for the work ahead, reflecting the pattern seen in creation itself — evening leading into morning, rest preceding activity.

Ultimately, living within God's rhythm of work and rest restores balance that modern life often erodes. It nurtures physical vitality, emotional stability, and spiritual clarity. It also serves as a foretaste of the ultimate rest promised in Christ, when striving will cease and renewal will be complete. Until then, each intentional pause becomes both a remembrance and a rehearsal — a reminder that human life was never meant to be sustained by relentless effort, but by trust in the God who renews His people day by day.

Sabbath as a Gift: Spiritual and Emotional Renewal

When God established the Sabbath, He framed it not as a burden but as a blessing. "The Sabbath was made for man," Jesus said in Mark 2:27, emphasizing that this rhythm was designed to serve humanity's well-being rather than impose unnecessary restriction. In a world that prizes constant productivity, this perspective is both liberating and countercultural. The Sabbath is an invitation to step out of the endless demands of life and receive rest, renewal, and deeper communion with God.

Spiritually, the Sabbath creates space to reconnect with the heart of faith. Work and daily responsibilities can easily crowd out reflection and prayer, leaving little room to remember God's presence. By intentionally setting aside time, believers open themselves to receive rather than strive. This posture transforms worship from obligation into delight. Time in Scripture feels less rushed, prayers become more attentive, and the soul regains a sense of alignment. The Sabbath reminds us that relationship with God is central to all other aspects of life and that rest is not merely physical recovery but spiritual recalibration.

The Sabbath also reorients perspective on identity. In a culture where worth is often tied to achievement, stopping work challenges the notion that value is earned. It declares that life and dignity are rooted in being children of God rather than in accomplishments. This shift fosters humility and gratitude, breaking the cycle of self-reliance. The weekly pause becomes a living testimony that God sustains life even when hands are still, and that joy does not depend on constant activity.

Emotional renewal is another vital gift of Sabbath. Human beings are not designed for unending stress. Without rest, anxiety compounds, relationships strain, and creativity diminishes. Observing a Sabbath rhythm interrupts this cycle, providing a structured opportunity to breathe and recover. It allows the nervous system to settle and the mind to refocus, offering relief from the noise of daily pressures. Over time, this rhythm of rest strengthens resilience, enabling believers to approach challenges with greater peace and clarity.

The Sabbath is also a time for delight. Biblical rest was not merely about ceasing from labor but about celebrating God's goodness. Meals were shared, songs were sung, and joy was cultivated. Reclaiming this celebratory aspect today can transform how rest is experienced. Rather than seeing it as simply "doing nothing," believers can view the Sabbath as a chance to savor blessings — enjoying nature, meaningful conversations, or creative pursuits that refresh the soul. This joyful dimension reinforces that rest is not only restorative but also deeply life-giving.

The communal nature of the Sabbath enriches its gift even further. In Scripture, it was not observed in isolation but shared among families and communities. This collective pause fostered a rhythm of togetherness, where meals, worship, and reflection became opportunities to deepen relationships. Modern life often fragments families and friendships through conflicting schedules and constant digital distraction. A shared day of rest can reclaim space for meaningful connection, where conversations flow without hurry and gratitude is practiced together. In this way, Sabbath rest becomes a relational sanctuary, nourishing not only the individual but also the bonds between people.

Practicing Sabbath in today's world requires intentionality rather than perfection. Few can replicate the quiet simplicity of ancient life, yet the principle of sacred pause is adaptable. Setting boundaries with technology, planning unhurried meals, or dedicating time for Scripture and prayer can establish a rhythm of rest even amid modern demands. The key is approaching it with purpose — choosing practices that genuinely foster renewal rather than defaulting to passive distraction. When done thoughtfully, these rhythms transform ordinary days into moments of holy restoration.

Embracing Sabbath also nurtures gratitude. By stepping back from constant striving, the heart gains perspective on blessings that might otherwise go unnoticed. The beauty of creation, the gift of relationships, and even the provision of daily needs become more apparent when given space to breathe. This gratitude spills over into the rest of the week, subtly reshaping how challenges are faced and how God's presence is recognized in the ordinary.

The Sabbath's role as a foretaste of eternity adds even greater depth. Scripture describes the ultimate rest awaiting God's people — a rest free from toil, suffering, and striving. Weekly rhythms of rest point toward this promise, reminding believers that life's burdens are temporary and that true renewal is found in Christ. Each Sabbath becomes a rehearsal for the future, a day that whispers of the coming restoration when all things will be made new.

Above all, receiving the Sabbath as a gift requires trust. It means believing that God's design for rest is not restrictive but life-giving, that stepping away from work will not lead to lack but to deeper abundance. This trust transforms rest from something earned to something received, shifting focus from human effort to divine provision. As this truth takes root, Sabbath moves from being an obligation to a joy — a rhythm that refreshes body, mind, and spirit, anchoring believers in the unchanging goodness of God.

Building Restorative Rhythms into a Busy Modern Life

Modern life rarely slows down. Work schedules bleed into personal time, notifications demand constant attention, and the pace of everyday responsibilities often feels relentless. Many people sense the need for rest but struggle to find a way to make it happen without falling behind. Building restorative rhythms into this kind of environment requires intentional choices — not just carving out occasional breaks, but reshaping daily and weekly patterns to align with God's design for balance.

The starting point is recognizing that rest is not simply the absence of work but the presence of renewal. Without this shift, attempts at rest often default to mindless distraction rather than true restoration. Scrolling through a phone or collapsing in front of a screen might offer temporary escape, yet it rarely leaves the heart or body refreshed. In contrast, biblical rest engages both body and soul. It invites reflection, gratitude, and a deeper awareness of God's presence in ordinary life.

Identifying natural points of transition in the day can help integrate this kind of rest. Short pauses before meals, brief moments of prayer upon waking or before sleep, or quiet walks during breaks can serve as anchors that recenter the mind. These moments do not require additional time so much as a reorientation of attention. By layering small practices of stillness into existing routines, renewal becomes part of the rhythm rather than an added burden.

Weekly patterns also play a crucial role. A dedicated Sabbath — whether a full day or a portion of a day — provides a reset that cannot be replicated by scattered moments of rest alone. Planning ahead makes this sustainable. Preparing meals in advance, finishing key tasks early, or setting boundaries with work communications can create the margin needed to enter rest fully. Over time, this rhythm becomes self-reinforcing; the body begins to anticipate the pause, and the mind learns to settle more easily into gratitude and worship.

Restorative rhythms also involve discernment in activity. Some practices that appear restful can actually drain energy, while others require effort yet restore deeply. For one person, gardening or cooking may be renewing; for another, reading Scripture in a quiet space might provide the greatest sense of peace. The goal is not to imitate someone else's routine but to discover what truly brings life and connection to God. Paying attention to how different activities impact emotional and physical energy can guide these choices, ensuring that rest aligns with personal needs and season of life.

Establishing these rhythms requires guarding boundaries that modern culture often erodes. Without intention, free time quickly fills with errands, obligations, or constant digital engagement. Setting clear limits — such as designated phone-free hours or defined work cutoffs — creates the space needed for true restoration. This is not about rigid rules but about creating freedom. Boundaries open the door for presence, allowing the heart to settle into gratitude instead of being pulled in every direction.

Community support can strengthen these commitments. Sharing rhythms with family or close friends fosters accountability and transforms rest from an individual pursuit into a shared experience. Planning simple weekly traditions — like a meal together, a walk in nature, or an evening of Scripture and prayer — reinforces connection while grounding life in values that outlast temporary busyness. These practices model to children and others in the home that rest is both valuable and normal, forming habits that carry into future generations.

Restorative rhythms also include listening to the body's signals. Fatigue, irritability, and lack of focus often indicate that rest is overdue. Ignoring these cues leads to deeper exhaustion and, over time, can manifest as physical illness or emotional burnout. Honoring these signals by slowing down, seeking prayer, or adjusting schedules reflects stewardship of the body God entrusted to us. Caring for physical well-being in this way is not selfish but an act of gratitude and preparation for continued service.

Incorporating creation into rest deepens its restorative impact. Time outdoors — whether sitting by water, walking through trees, or simply observing the sky — shifts perspective and invites awe. These moments often quiet inner noise and remind believers of God's presence in the natural world. Creation itself reflects His rhythm of work and rest, from the cycles of day and night to the changing of seasons. Aligning personal rhythms with this design fosters peace that artificial environments rarely provide.

Ultimately, building restorative rhythms is about trust. It is trusting that God can sustain what we release during our moments of rest, that productivity does not define worth, and that peace flows from alignment with His design rather than relentless effort. Over time, these practices reorient life away from frantic striving toward steady dependence on God's presence. Rest becomes more than a break; it becomes a way of living — a quiet strength that carries into work, relationships, and worship alike.

Part III. Healing the Mind and Spirit

Physical renewal is important, but Scripture reminds us that true wholeness reaches deeper than the body. Many of life's struggles begin not in muscles or bones but in the unseen places of thought, belief, and emotion. The heart and mind shape how we experience the world, how we respond to suffering, and even how we engage with God. When these inner places are wounded or burdened, outward health often suffers as well.

The Bible speaks to this reality with profound clarity. It describes the mind as a battlefield, a space where lies, fears, and anxieties contend with faith and truth. It calls believers to "be transformed by the renewing of your mind" and to guard their hearts, knowing that life flows from them. These words point to an inseparable link between inner healing and outer well-being, revealing that care for the soul is not optional but essential.

Modern research echoes this connection. Studies in psychology and neuroscience confirm what Scripture has long proclaimed: chronic stress, unresolved trauma, and negative thought patterns can contribute to physical illness and emotional instability. Conversely, practices that foster gratitude, hope, and forgiveness promote resilience and even measurable improvements in health. This harmony between biblical wisdom and scientific insight underscores God's intricate design — a design in which body, mind, and spirit are deeply interwoven.

In this part of the book, we turn our attention to this inner landscape. We will explore themes of renewing the mind through Scripture, breaking free from toxic thoughts, cultivating peace in the midst of anxiety, and rediscovering joy through trust in God's promises. These chapters are not about quick fixes but about building patterns of thought and prayer that invite lasting transformation. They will guide you in integrating spiritual truths with practical tools, offering a pathway to healing that honors both faith and wisdom.

Approaching this journey requires patience and honesty. Inner wounds do not heal overnight, and meaningful change often begins in small, hidden ways. Yet the promise of Scripture is sure: God draws near to the brokenhearted, binds up their wounds, and offers peace that surpasses understanding. Healing the mind and spirit is not about striving harder but about opening ourselves to the One who restores us from within.

Chapter 7: Prayer and Meditation for Healing

Praying the Psalms: Words of Comfort and Strength

The Psalms have served as the prayer book of God's people for centuries, offering words that bridge the gap between human experience and divine presence. Their enduring power lies in their honesty. They do not gloss over pain or pretend life is always orderly. Instead, they give voice to raw emotions — sorrow, joy, fear, gratitude, longing — and invite believers to bring these emotions before God. This openness makes the Psalms especially powerful for those seeking comfort and strength in difficult seasons.

Many people struggle to find the right words when they pray, especially in times of suffering or confusion. The Psalms meet this need by providing language already shaped by the Spirit and affirmed by Scripture. Praying them allows believers to borrow the words of David, Asaph, and other psalmists when their own words feel inadequate. These prayers remind us that we are not alone in our struggles; countless generations have lifted the same cries, rejoiced in the same promises, and found peace in the same God.

The Psalms encompass a remarkable breadth of human experience. Laments like Psalm 13 capture the ache of waiting for God's deliverance: "How long, Lord? Will you forget me forever?" In contrast, songs of thanksgiving like Psalm 103 overflow with praise: "Bless the Lord, O my soul, and forget not all his benefits." This range allows believers to approach God authentically, whether they are celebrating victories or wrestling with unanswered questions. There is no emotion too dark or too joyful to bring into His presence.

Praying the Psalms also trains the heart to see beyond immediate circumstances. Many psalms begin with despair but end in trust, moving from complaint to confidence. This pattern reflects a journey of faith: acknowledging pain honestly, yet choosing to anchor hope in God's character rather than in changing circumstances. As these words are prayed repeatedly, they form habits of resilience, teaching the soul to cling to truth even when feelings waver.

Modern studies on mental and emotional health affirm the benefits of this kind of honest, structured prayer. Research by Dr. Kenneth Pargament in 2013, for example, highlights how spiritual practices rooted in sacred texts reduce anxiety and foster meaning in adversity. While science describes the outcomes, Scripture reveals the source — communion with a God who listens and responds. The Psalms offer not only comfort but transformation, reshaping how believers think and feel as they engage with God's promises.

In practical terms, praying the Psalms can be deeply personal. Some read them aloud each morning, using them as a framework for their own prayers. Others journal through them, rewriting verses in their own words as a way of processing emotion. Still others sing them, following the psalmists' original intent as songs of worship. The form matters less than the posture — approaching God with openness and allowing His Word to guide both lament and praise.

The Psalms also invite believers to worship in every circumstance, not only when life feels secure or victories are evident. Psalm 34 declares, "I will bless the Lord at all times; His praise shall continually be in my mouth." Praying this verse in seasons of hardship challenges the heart to shift focus from what is lacking to the constancy of God's presence. This discipline does not deny pain but reframes it in light of His faithfulness, cultivating peace even in uncertainty.

In times of fear or anxiety, the Psalms become a refuge. Psalm 46 proclaims, "God is our refuge and strength, an ever-present help in trouble." Speaking these words aloud anchors faith in God's protection, especially when external circumstances feel overwhelming. Many believers find that repeating such verses during moments of stress helps quiet racing thoughts and reestablish calm. Over time, these prayers shape reflexive trust, so that turning to God becomes the first response rather than the last resort.

Communal prayer is another dimension of the Psalms' power. Originally sung in temple worship and later in synagogues and churches, these texts were designed to unite God's people in shared devotion. Praying them together today — in families, small groups, or congregations — deepens connection and reminds individuals that they are part of a larger story. In suffering, collective lament brings comfort; in celebration, shared praise magnifies joy. This corporate aspect reflects the Psalms' enduring role in shaping the spiritual identity of God's people.

Personalizing the Psalms can also deepen their impact. While the words remain timeless, inserting specific names, situations, or emotions helps apply them directly to present circumstances. A verse about deliverance can be prayed over a struggling loved one; a line of thanksgiving can be spoken in gratitude for specific blessings. This practice transforms the Psalms from ancient poetry into living prayers that speak directly to the challenges and joys of modern life.

Engaging the Psalms consistently cultivates resilience. Their cadence of lament and praise mirrors the rhythms of human experience, normalizing the ebb and flow of emotions in the life of faith. As believers return to these prayers over weeks and months, they often discover verses becoming part of memory, ready to surface in moments of need. A whispered line from Psalm 23 or Psalm 91 can provide comfort in hospital rooms, at gravesides, or during sleepless nights, carrying God's promises into the darkest places.

Ultimately, the gift of the Psalms lies in their capacity to draw believers closer to God in honesty and trust. They affirm that every feeling — joy, fear, anger, longing — can be brought before Him without shame. In praying them, the heart learns to rest in His character rather than in fluctuating circumstances. Over time, these prayers become more than words; they become a lifeline, anchoring the soul in God's unchanging love and providing comfort and strength for every season of life.

Scripture Meditation: Renewing the Mind and Spirit

Meditating on Scripture is one of the most transformative practices in the life of faith. Unlike casual reading, meditation invites the Word to dwell deeply, shaping thought patterns and renewing the heart from the inside out. It is not about rushing through chapters or checking off a reading plan, but about slowing down enough for truth to penetrate the layers of distraction and worry that often cloud the mind. Through meditation, Scripture moves from information to formation, gradually aligning beliefs and responses with God's heart.

The Bible itself calls believers to this practice repeatedly. Psalm 1 describes the blessed person as one who delights in the law of the Lord and meditates on it day and night, comparing them to a tree planted by streams of water — rooted, nourished, and fruitful. Joshua 1:8 commands meditation on the Book of the Law as the key to success and prosperity, not in material terms but in the flourishing that comes from living aligned with God's will. These passages reveal that meditation is not optional but central to spiritual health, a rhythm as vital as prayer or worship.

In practical terms, meditation means lingering with a passage, turning it over in the mind, and allowing its meaning to sink deep. This often involves repetition — reading a verse slowly several times, emphasizing different words, or quietly reciting it in prayer. Some find it helpful to picture the imagery Scripture offers, such as imagining themselves lying down in green pastures in Psalm 23 or standing still as waves of peace wash over them in Isaiah 26:3. Others focus on a single phrase, letting it echo throughout the day as a quiet anchor amid busyness.

The renewal that comes from this practice is both subtle and profound. Over time, meditation reshapes thought patterns, gently replacing anxiety with trust and discouragement with hope. Modern neuroscience even affirms this process: studies on focused reflection and mindfulness show measurable changes in the brain, reducing stress and increasing emotional resilience. While biblical meditation differs in its God-centered focus, it similarly cultivates calm and clarity — not through self-emptying, but by filling the mind with truth.

Meditation also strengthens the connection between mind and heart. It moves Scripture from being abstract knowledge into lived reality. Reading that God is faithful is one thing; sitting quietly with that truth, recalling His faithfulness in personal experience, is another. This deeper engagement builds confidence in His promises and fosters intimacy with Him. The more time spent reflecting on His Word, the more naturally it comes to mind in moments of need, offering guidance and comfort without conscious effort.

As meditation becomes a consistent rhythm, it begins to transform daily life in quiet but profound ways. The words stored in the heart provide stability in moments of stress, offering reassurance when anxiety rises or decisions weigh heavily. A verse repeated throughout the day can shift the tone of an entire situation, not by changing circumstances but by reframing how they are experienced. This subtle reorientation helps the believer remain anchored in God's truth even when emotions fluctuate. Scripture meditation also cultivates patience in a culture of hurry. Modern life conditions people to expect instant results, but the work of renewal happens gradually. Allowing the Word to take root requires trust in God's timing. Like seeds planted in soil, the truths of Scripture germinate unseen before bearing fruit. This process fosters humility, teaching reliance on God rather than quick fixes or self-effort. Over time, the fruit of this practice — peace, clarity, resilience — becomes evident to both the individual and those around them.

Another benefit is the deepening of prayer life. Meditation naturally flows into conversation with God. As verses are reflected upon, they spark gratitude, confession, and intercession. A promise about God's presence might lead to thanksgiving; a verse about forgiveness may prompt honest confession. In this way, meditation and prayer intertwine, creating a dialogue that moves beyond formal words into an ongoing awareness of God throughout the day.

Practical approaches can make meditation accessible even amid busy schedules. Beginning with a single verse or short passage can be more effective than trying to cover long sections. Writing the verse on a card or setting it as a phone reminder keeps it present during daily routines. Morning and evening are natural entry points — starting the day with grounding truth and ending it with reflection fosters continuity. Over time, this simple rhythm develops into a habit that shapes the entire day. The goal of meditation is not perfection but presence. There will be days when focus wavers or distractions intrude, yet even these imperfect moments can become opportunities to return to God. Each act of refocusing is itself a form of prayer, a quiet turning of the heart toward the One who invites continual communion. As this practice deepens, Scripture becomes less a text to study and more a living voice guiding, comforting, and renewing every aspect of life.

Ultimately, meditating on God's Word is about more than personal peace. It equips believers to live differently — to respond with grace under pressure, to extend compassion in conflict, and to anchor their identity in God's promises rather than shifting circumstances. This inner renewal overflows outward, influencing relationships, work, and the way challenges are faced. By allowing Scripture to dwell richly within, the believer steps into the life God intended: steady, rooted, and continually refreshed by the streams of His living Word.

Creating a Daily Prayer Rhythm That Supports Wholeness

Prayer is more than a spiritual discipline; it is a lifeline that connects believers to the heart of God. While spontaneous prayers have their place, Scripture and Christian tradition both reveal the value of intentional rhythms — set times of prayer that anchor the day and keep the heart aligned with God's presence. In a culture driven by urgency and distraction, establishing these rhythms offers a steady foundation for emotional, mental, and spiritual health.

The concept of regular prayer is rooted in Scripture itself. The psalmist declares, "Evening, morning, and noon I cry out in distress, and He hears my voice" (Psalm 55:17). Daniel is described as praying three times a day, even under threat of persecution. These examples show that structured prayer was not a constraint but a source of strength, providing focus and continuity in every season of life. It recognized the truth that just as the body needs consistent nourishment, the soul needs consistent communion with God.

Creating a daily rhythm begins with understanding its purpose. Prayer is not about reciting words to fulfill a duty but about cultivating awareness of God's presence throughout the day. A rhythm serves as a reminder to pause, breathe, and realign with His truth amid the demands of work, relationships, and responsibilities. Over time, these pauses transform how challenges are faced and how blessings are received, infusing ordinary moments with sacred meaning.

One practical approach is to anchor prayer to natural transitions in the day. Morning prayer sets intention and frames the day with gratitude and dependence on God. Midday prayer offers a moment to recalibrate, especially when fatigue or stress begins to build. Evening prayer invites reflection, confession, and rest in God's care. This pattern need not be complicated; even a few minutes of focused prayer at each point can cultivate stability and peace.

The content of these prayers can vary depending on personal needs and circumstances. Mornings may focus on surrender and guidance: asking God to lead in decisions and interactions. Midday prayers might center on strength and perspective, lifting ongoing challenges and offering thanks for small victories. Evenings can invite reflection, reviewing the day with God, acknowledging failures without condemnation, and celebrating moments of grace. Over time, these rhythms build a habit of living prayerfully, where conversation with God flows naturally into every part of life.

Sustaining a daily rhythm of prayer also involves creating an environment that encourages consistency. A dedicated space, even something as simple as a quiet corner or a chair by a window, can serve as a physical reminder to pause. Some keep a journal or Bible in this space, ready to capture prayers and insights. These tangible cues signal the mind and heart to slow down and enter into conversation with God. Over time, the space itself becomes associated with peace and stillness, making it easier to return even on busy days.

Flexibility is essential to keeping this rhythm life-giving rather than burdensome. Life seasons change, and so do schedules. What matters is not rigid adherence but faithful return. A parent caring for young children may find brief prayers throughout the day more realistic than long periods of stillness. Someone with demanding work may choose early mornings or late evenings for extended time with God. The rhythm is meant to serve the person, not the other way around, and God honors the heart that seeks Him, whether through whispered prayers or structured times of silence.

Integrating Scripture into these prayer times deepens their impact. Praying through passages, such as the Lord's Prayer or a psalm, provides a framework when words are hard to find and ensures alignment with God's truth. Many find it helpful to focus on a single verse or theme each week, allowing it to guide their prayers and thoughts throughout the day. This approach transforms prayer from a task into an ongoing dialogue shaped by God's Word rather than personal anxieties alone.

Community can enrich personal rhythms as well. Sharing prayer commitments with a friend or family member provides encouragement and accountability. Some choose to begin or end the day praying together, while others exchange brief messages or calls to check in and support one another. These connections remind believers that prayer is not only personal but also communal, drawing strength from the shared faith of others.

The long-term fruit of daily prayer rhythms often becomes evident gradually. Over weeks and months, many notice a growing sense of steadiness, a greater ability to handle stress, and a deeper awareness of God's presence in ordinary life. Challenges remain, but the way they are carried shifts; prayer transforms burdens into opportunities for trust and dependence. This quiet resilience becomes a testimony to those around, revealing a life anchored not in perfect circumstances but in consistent communion with God.

Ultimately, establishing a daily prayer rhythm is about aligning life with God's presence rather than fitting Him into the margins. It is about cultivating an ongoing awareness that shapes decisions, relationships, and responses to challenges. As these rhythms deepen, prayer moves from being something scheduled to something lived — a steady current beneath the surface of daily life that renews mind, body, and spirit and draws the believer into closer fellowship with the One who sustains all things.

Chapter 8: Forgiveness and Emotional Restoration

The Healing Power of Forgiveness in Scripture

Forgiveness is one of the most radical and transformative themes in Scripture. It touches the deepest wounds of the human heart and offers a pathway not only to reconciliation with others but also to personal healing. While the world often views forgiveness as optional or conditional, the Bible presents it as central to the life of faith — a reflection of God's own character and a key to experiencing freedom from bitterness and emotional pain.

From the earliest pages of Scripture, forgiveness is woven into the story of God's people. Joseph's response to his brothers in Genesis 50 is one of the most striking examples. Betrayed, sold into slavery, and left for dead, Joseph eventually rose to power in Egypt. When his brothers came seeking help during a famine, he had every reason to retaliate. Instead, he forgave, declaring, "You meant evil against me, but God meant it for good." This perspective — seeing beyond personal hurt to God's redemptive purposes — illustrates the depth of biblical forgiveness. It is not denial of wrong but a choice to release vengeance and trust God with justice.

Jesus' teaching elevates forgiveness even further, making it central to the kingdom of God. In the Sermon on the Mount, He instructs His followers to pray, "Forgive us our debts, as we also have forgiven our debtors" (Matthew 6:12). This prayer links receiving forgiveness from God with extending it to others, emphasizing that grace received must become grace given. The parable of the unforgiving servant underscores this point vividly, revealing the hypocrisy of accepting mercy yet refusing to extend it. For Jesus, forgiveness is not optional but an essential expression of love and obedience.

Forgiveness in Scripture also has profound implications for emotional and physical health. Modern research confirms what biblical wisdom has long suggested: harboring resentment increases stress, disrupts sleep, and can even contribute to cardiovascular problems. Conversely, forgiving others has been shown to lower anxiety, reduce depression, and promote overall well-being. While forgiveness does not erase the memory of harm, it releases the hold that pain and anger can have over the heart. In this sense, forgiving is as much about personal healing as it is about restoring relationships.

Yet forgiveness is often misunderstood. It is not excusing harmful behavior, minimizing pain, or forgetting what happened. Nor is it necessarily reconciliation, which requires repentance and rebuilding trust. Forgiveness, in its biblical sense, is a decision to release someone from the debt they owe, entrusting ultimate justice to God. This distinction is critical because it frees the injured person from carrying the weight of the offense without placing them in harm's way. Forgiveness is a gift to both the offender and the one forgiving, a step toward freedom that refuses to let bitterness define the future.

Choosing to forgive can be one of the hardest decisions a person makes, especially when the wound is deep. Scripture acknowledges this struggle. Jesus' command to forgive "seventy times seven" was not about keeping count but about cultivating a posture of continual grace. This requires surrender — releasing the desire for revenge and entrusting the outcome to God's justice and mercy. Such forgiveness may not happen instantly; it is often a process of repeatedly bringing the pain before God and allowing Him to soften the heart over time.

The act of forgiving transforms the one who forgives as much as it impacts the one being forgiven. It interrupts cycles of anger and frees the soul from the burden of carrying resentment. Many who choose forgiveness describe an unexpected sense of peace, even if the relationship itself remains unreconciled. This peace is not born of forgetting what happened but from laying down the need to repay hurt for hurt. In this way, forgiveness becomes a form of healing prayer, inviting God to mend what human strength cannot.

Jesus modeled this powerfully on the cross. As He endured unimaginable suffering, He prayed, "Father, forgive them, for they know not what they do" (Luke 23:34). This prayer captures the heart of biblical forgiveness:

interceding for those who cause harm and entrusting them to God's mercy. His example shows that forgiveness is not limited by the magnitude of the offense. If Christ could extend grace to those crucifying Him, His followers are invited to reflect that same grace in their own lives, relying on His strength rather than their own.

Practical steps toward forgiveness often begin with honest acknowledgment of pain. Denying or suppressing hurt only deepens resentment. Bringing these feelings into prayer — naming the offense before God, expressing anger, grief, or confusion — creates space for healing to begin. From there, the choice to release the offender becomes possible, even if feelings lag behind. Forgiveness is both a moment and a journey; it may need to be reaffirmed many times before the heart fully aligns with the decision.

Forgiveness also invites reflection on the forgiveness believers themselves have received. Remembering the weight of one's own debt before God fosters humility and compassion toward others. The parable of the prodigal son illustrates this dynamic beautifully: the father's embrace of the wayward son reflects God's boundless mercy and challenges His people to extend similar grace. This perspective does not minimize wrongdoing but situates it within the larger story of divine forgiveness that covers every believer.

The fruit of forgiveness extends beyond the individual to communities and relationships. Families fractured by conflict can begin to heal when even one member chooses grace. Friendships can be restored, and churches can model reconciliation to a divided world. Forgiveness does not erase all consequences, but it opens the door to peace — peace within the heart and peace in relationships where healing is possible.

Ultimately, forgiveness is an act of trust. It entrusts the pain, the offender, and the outcome into God's hands, believing that His justice and mercy are perfect. In choosing to forgive, believers step into the freedom Christ offers, breaking free from the chains of bitterness and opening themselves to the healing only He can bring.

Releasing Bitterness: Biblical Practices for Inner Peace

Bitterness often begins quietly. A single wound, left unaddressed, can grow into lingering resentment that colors how we see ourselves, others, and even God. Over time, bitterness drains energy, clouds judgment, and disrupts relationships. Scripture speaks clearly about this danger: "See to it that no root of bitterness springs up and causes trouble, and by it many become defiled" (Hebrews 12:15). This imagery of a root is striking, for bitterness rarely stays hidden; it spreads, taking hold of the heart and influencing every part of life.

The Bible offers a path to freedom from this cycle. Releasing bitterness is not about pretending harm never happened or silencing the pain of injustice. It is about allowing God's grace to heal what bitterness has poisoned and choosing peace over the corrosive pull of resentment. This process is deeply personal yet profoundly transformative, requiring both honest self-examination and practical steps rooted in Scripture.

One of the first steps is recognizing bitterness when it surfaces. It often reveals itself through recurring thoughts about a person or event, difficulty celebrating others' blessings, or persistent anger that flares in unrelated situations. The Psalms provide language for this recognition, modeling raw honesty before God. David does not hide his anguish; he pours it out in prayer, expressing frustration and pleading for justice. This transparency is not weakness but the beginning of healing, as bringing bitterness into God's light allows Him to address it at its root.

Confession is another crucial practice. Bitterness may begin with legitimate hurt, but holding onto it can lead to sin — harsh words, judgmental attitudes, or a hardened heart. Admitting these responses before God opens the door to His cleansing and renewal. First John 1:9 assures that if we confess our sins, He is faithful to forgive and purify. Confession does not excuse the harm done by others; rather, it acknowledges our own need for grace and aligns us with God's heart for restoration.

Prayer for those who have caused pain is perhaps the most challenging yet liberating step. Jesus commands His followers to pray for their enemies, not to condone wrongdoing but to free the heart from hatred.

This prayer often begins reluctantly. Many find themselves praying for the willingness to forgive long before they feel compassion. Over time, consistent prayer softens the grip of bitterness, shifting focus from the offender's actions to God's ability to heal and redeem.

Gratitude serves as a powerful antidote to bitterness. Focusing on God's blessings reorients the heart away from what was lost or taken and toward what remains and is continually given. The Psalms frequently pair lament with thanksgiving, demonstrating that even amid sorrow there is room for praise. Practicing gratitude does not minimize pain; rather, it creates space for hope and invites God's presence into wounded places. Over time, gratitude reshapes perspective, making peace possible even when circumstances remain unresolved.

Community support is another vital element in this process. Bitterness thrives in isolation, where thoughts go unchallenged and hurt festers. Sharing struggles with trusted believers provides both accountability and encouragement. Scripture calls the body of Christ to "bear one another's burdens," reminding us that healing often unfolds in relationship. Wise counsel, prayer partners, and supportive fellowship can help identify blind spots and reinforce the commitment to release resentment when old memories resurface.

Replacing bitterness with compassion is the final movement toward lasting peace. This shift does not happen through sheer willpower but through encountering God's compassion for ourselves. As His mercy becomes more real, it naturally flows toward others, even those who have caused harm. This transformation is described vividly in Ephesians 4:31-32: "Get rid of all bitterness, rage and anger... Be kind and compassionate to one another, forgiving each other, just as in Christ God forgave you." Here, forgiveness and compassion are inseparable, rooted not in what others deserve but in what God has already done.

The freedom that follows release is profound. Those who let go of bitterness often describe a weight lifting, an inner stillness replacing constant tension. This peace is not dependent on reconciliation or apology; it is anchored in trusting God with justice and embracing His invitation to live unbound. Freed from the burden of resentment, the heart becomes open again to joy, to love, and to deeper intimacy with God.

Releasing bitterness is ultimately a journey of surrender. It requires courage to face pain honestly, humility to seek God's help, and perseverance to return to Him whenever old wounds resurface. Yet the promise of Scripture is clear: those who release bitterness will experience peace that surpasses understanding. By practicing confession, prayer, gratitude, and compassion, believers align their hearts with God's healing work and step into the freedom He longs for them to know.

Restoring Relationships Through Grace and Reconciliation

Broken relationships are among the deepest sources of human pain. Whether caused by betrayal, misunderstanding, or neglect, fractured connections leave emotional scars that can linger for years. Scripture acknowledges this reality and does not minimize the hurt, yet it continually calls believers toward reconciliation wherever possible. At the heart of this call is grace — the undeserved favor God extends to humanity, which His people are invited to reflect toward one another.

Grace begins with recognizing our own need for it. The apostle Paul reminds us in Romans 3:23 that all have sinned and fall short of God's glory. This truth levels the ground, dismantling the illusion of moral superiority and softening the heart toward others. When believers grasp the magnitude of the grace they have received, they are better equipped to extend that grace, even to those who have wounded them. Reconciliation, then, becomes less about tallying faults and more about responding to God's mercy.

Biblical reconciliation is more than a polite truce or avoidance of conflict; it seeks restoration of trust and unity wherever it can be safely pursued. Jesus' teaching in Matthew 5 underscores this priority, urging His followers to seek reconciliation even before offering gifts at the altar. This reveals how central healed relationships are to worship and spiritual life. Pursuing reconciliation honors God's design for community and reflects the reconciling work of Christ, who bridges the ultimate divide between humanity and God.

The process often begins with honest self-examination. Before approaching another person, Scripture calls believers to examine their own hearts — acknowledging personal faults, confessing pride, and discerning whether their desire for reconciliation flows from love rather than from a need to prove a point. Jesus' teaching about removing the plank from one's own eye before addressing the speck in another's illustrates this principle. True reconciliation cannot happen without humility and a willingness to see one's own contribution to the conflict.

Taking the first step is often the hardest part. Fear of rejection or reopening old wounds can feel paralyzing, yet Scripture repeatedly calls for initiative. Romans 12:18 encourages believers to live at peace with everyone "as far as it depends on you." This does not guarantee reconciliation, as it requires mutual willingness, but it does mean taking responsibility for the part within one's control. A simple gesture — a letter, a conversation, or an apology — can begin to dismantle walls built over time.

Reconciliation unfolds best when approached with a spirit of listening rather than accusation. Creating space to hear the other person's perspective — even when it is difficult — honors their dignity and opens the door for mutual understanding. This does not mean agreeing with everything said but being willing to understand the emotions behind it. Many conflicts soften not through winning arguments but through the healing that comes when someone feels genuinely heard and valued.

Grace also guides the way conversations are framed. Speaking truth is important, yet Scripture calls for it to be done in love. Harsh words may satisfy momentary frustration but rarely lead to lasting peace. Choosing gentleness does not deny the reality of hurt; it simply prioritizes restoration over retaliation. This approach mirrors Christ's ministry, where firm truth was always coupled with compassion, drawing people toward transformation rather than driving them away.

Forgiveness plays a vital role in restoring trust, though it does not always mean immediate restoration of the relationship to what it once was. Boundaries may still be necessary, especially in cases of ongoing harm or unrepentance. Forgiveness releases the grip of resentment; reconciliation, when possible, rebuilds mutual respect and trust over time. Both are rooted in grace, but reconciliation is a journey that requires patience and sometimes professional or pastoral support.

When reconciliation succeeds, the impact ripples outward. Families once divided can begin to heal, friendships can be renewed, and communities can witness the power of God's love at work. This restoration testifies to the gospel itself, for at its core, the Christian message is about reconciliation — God making peace with humanity through Christ and calling His people to be ministers of that same reconciliation in the world.

There are times, however, when reconciliation is not possible, whether due to safety, unwillingness, or circumstances beyond control. Even then, grace remains essential. Choosing peace in one's own heart, praying for the other person, and entrusting the unresolved situation to God allows healing to continue even without mutual restoration. The goal is not to force an outcome but to walk faithfully, reflecting God's character in every step.

Living out reconciliation requires courage and perseverance, yet it brings profound freedom. It frees the heart from bitterness, softens hardened places, and restores the joy that resentment often steals. More than that, it mirrors the very nature of God, whose grace mends what is broken and whose love makes all things new. When believers choose reconciliation, they participate in this divine work, becoming vessels of peace in a fractured world and living out the gospel they profess.

Chapter 9: Stress, Anxiety, and Peace of Mind

"Do Not Be Anxious": What the Bible Teaches About Worry

Anxiety is a universal human experience. It arises from uncertainty about the future, fear of loss, or the weight of responsibilities that feel beyond control. In Scripture, God speaks repeatedly to this condition of the heart, not with condemnation but with reassurance. The repeated command, "Do not be anxious," found in passages like Philippians 4:6 and Matthew 6:25, is not a demand to suppress feelings but an invitation to trust — to shift focus from personal striving to God's faithful care.

Jesus' teaching in the Sermon on the Mount addresses worry with remarkable clarity. He points to the birds of the air and the lilies of the field, neither of which labor or store away, yet are sustained and clothed by the Father. His conclusion is both comforting and challenging: "Are you not much more valuable than they?" (Matthew 6:26). This question reframes anxiety, reminding believers that God's care is both personal and intentional. If creation itself is tended so carefully, how much more will He provide for His children?

Paul's words in Philippians 4 build on this foundation. "Do not be anxious about anything," he writes, "but in every situation, by prayer and petition, with thanksgiving, present your requests to God." This verse does not deny the reality of anxious thoughts; it offers a practical alternative. Anxiety is countered through prayer — not a single prayer uttered once, but a posture of continual dialogue with God. Gratitude is woven into this practice, redirecting attention from what is lacking to what has already been given. The result is described as "the peace of God, which transcends all understanding," a peace that guards both heart and mind.

This biblical perspective challenges the cultural narrative that equates peace with control. Modern approaches to worry often focus on managing circumstances — planning more, preparing harder, predicting outcomes. While wisdom and planning have their place, Scripture points to a deeper truth: lasting peace flows not from mastering the future but from trusting the One who holds it. This shift in perspective does not remove difficulty but anchors the believer in stability that circumstances cannot shake.

The call to release anxiety also acknowledges human limitation. Psalm 127 reminds us, "In vain you rise early and stay up late, toiling for food to eat — for He grants sleep to those He loves." Rest, both physical and spiritual, is a gift from God, not an achievement of effort. Embracing this gift requires humility — a willingness to admit that we are not self-sufficient and that dependence on God is not weakness but wisdom.

One of the most powerful truths Scripture offers about anxiety is God's nearness. Philippians 4:5 precedes the well-known verse about prayer with this assurance: "The Lord is near." This closeness is not symbolic; it is a promise that God walks with His people through every fear and uncertainty. Anxiety often magnifies isolation, convincing the heart that it must face struggles alone. Recalling God's presence breaks this illusion, bringing comfort that circumstances alone cannot provide.

Another layer of biblical teaching on worry is the focus on today rather than tomorrow. Jesus' words in Matthew 6:34 — "Do not worry about tomorrow, for tomorrow will worry about itself" — call attention to the futility of projecting fear into the future. Worry multiplies imagined outcomes, many of which never come to pass. By anchoring attention in the present, believers learn to trust God for daily provision rather than demanding a full view of what lies ahead. This shift encourages living in step with grace given for each moment rather than being crushed under the weight of imagined burdens.

Scripture also invites believers to replace anxious thoughts with truths about God's character. Isaiah 26:3 declares, "You will keep in perfect peace those whose minds are steadfast, because they trust in You." This steadfastness is cultivated by rehearsing what is true: God's goodness, His promises, His past faithfulness. When the mind is saturated with these realities, anxiety loses its power to dominate. This practice does not deny problems but reframes them in light of a God who is bigger than every fear.

Practical application flows from these truths. Building habits of prayerful reflection throughout the day interrupts cycles of worry before they spiral. Simple pauses to breathe, recite a verse, or thank God for His presence create moments of reset. Over time, these habits form new neural pathways, teaching the mind to turn first toward trust rather than fear. This aligns with both biblical teaching and modern understanding of how repeated practices can reshape thought patterns and emotional responses.

The process of learning not to be anxious is gradual. It requires patience with oneself and reliance on God's Spirit, who empowers change from within. There will be moments when worry resurfaces, but each return to prayer is another act of trust, another reminder that God's peace is available. With practice, the heart grows more attuned to His presence, and worry loosens its grip.

Ultimately, the command not to be anxious is less about what to avoid and more about what to embrace — faith in a God who sees, provides, and sustains. Trusting Him does not remove challenges, but it transforms how they are carried. In this trust, believers find rest that the world cannot offer: a deep, enduring peace rooted not in circumstances but in the unchanging character of God.

Trust and Surrender: Healing Through Faith

Trusting God is one of the most profound yet challenging aspects of spiritual life. It requires letting go of control, releasing the need to predict outcomes, and believing that God's plans are good even when they are unclear. In Scripture, this trust is inseparable from surrender — the act of yielding our fears, ambitions, and burdens to Him. Together, trust and surrender form the foundation for deep healing, offering peace that transcends understanding and strength for the trials of life.

The call to trust God is woven throughout the Bible. Proverbs 3:5-6 captures it simply yet powerfully: "Trust in the Lord with all your heart and lean not on your own understanding; in all your ways submit to Him, and He will make your paths straight." This verse challenges the natural instinct to rely on personal insight or control. It invites believers to place confidence in God's wisdom, acknowledging that His perspective spans past, present, and future in ways human vision cannot.

Surrender often begins where self-sufficiency ends. Many turn to God most fully in moments of crisis — when resources are depleted, plans have failed, or pain feels unbearable. While surrender in these moments can be difficult, it also opens the door to profound encounters with God's faithfulness. Scripture offers numerous examples of this posture: Hannah releasing her longing for a child, David entrusting his life to God while pursued by enemies, and Jesus in Gethsemane praying, "Not my will, but Yours be done." These stories reveal that surrender is not passive resignation but active trust, choosing God's way even when it is costly.

The connection between trust, surrender, and healing is deeply spiritual yet also practical. Anxiety, bitterness, and fear often thrive on the illusion of control. When believers release this need to manage every outcome, they create space for God's peace to take root. Modern research supports this biblical principle: studies in psychology show that relinquishing control and embracing trust — particularly in a higher power — reduces stress and promotes emotional well-being. This harmony between faith and evidence underscores the wisdom of Scripture's call to trust.

Yet trust and surrender do not come easily. They require intentional cultivation, built through prayer, reflection on God's promises, and recalling His past faithfulness. As believers look back on times when God has provided, guided, or sustained them, their confidence grows for present and future challenges. This remembrance transforms trust from an abstract concept into a lived reality, making surrender a natural response rather than a forced choice.

Trust deepens as believers encounter God's presence in daily life. Small acts of surrender — releasing worries in prayer, choosing to obey even when uncertain, acknowledging His hand in both blessings and challenges — create a pattern of dependence. Over time, this pattern transforms the way difficulties are experienced. Hardships may remain, but the heart carries them differently, anchored in the assurance that nothing is wasted in God's hands.

Surrender also reshapes priorities. When life is yielded to God, success is no longer measured by control or achievement but by faithfulness and alignment with His will. This shift relieves the constant pressure to manage outcomes and instead fosters freedom to live fully in the present. It becomes possible to pursue goals with diligence yet hold them loosely, trusting that God's plan, even when unexpected, leads to deeper good than personal striving could accomplish.

An important aspect of this process is honest communication with God. Surrender does not require suppressing fear or doubt; it welcomes bringing them into prayer. The Psalms model this beautifully, blending cries for help with declarations of trust. This authenticity builds intimacy with God, reminding believers that surrender is not about perfection but about relationship. It is choosing to trust Him with what is real — hopes, disappointments, confusion — and allowing His Spirit to bring comfort and clarity.

Community can play a supportive role in this journey. Walking alongside others who are learning to trust and surrender provides encouragement and perspective. Hearing testimonies of God's faithfulness strengthens faith and helps recalibrate focus when anxiety resurfaces. The body of Christ is designed to bear one another's burdens, making the process of surrender less isolating and more attainable.

The fruit of trust and surrender is profound peace. Philippians 4:7 describes it as a peace that "transcends all understanding," guarding hearts and minds in Christ Jesus. This peace is not dependent on the absence of trials but on the presence of God within them. It allows believers to navigate uncertainty with steadiness, to endure pain with hope, and to face the unknown with quiet confidence.

Ultimately, healing through faith comes as the heart learns to rest in God's sovereignty. Trust and surrender form a cycle: the more one surrenders, the deeper trust grows, and the deeper the trust, the easier it becomes to surrender again. In this rhythm, burdens are exchanged for rest, fear gives way to hope, and the soul finds renewal in the hands of the One who never fails.

Practical Tools to Reduce Stress and Restore Calm

Stress is unavoidable in modern life, but how we respond to it can either erode peace or strengthen resilience. Scripture repeatedly calls believers to live from a place of trust and calm, yet it also recognizes the real pressures people face daily. Bridging faith with practical steps allows this biblical vision of peace to become tangible, helping individuals move beyond momentary relief into lasting stability of mind and spirit.

One of the most effective ways to address stress is through intentional breathing and stillness. The Bible frequently portrays quietness as a posture of trust — "Be still, and know that I am God" (Psalm 46:10). Taking even a few minutes to pause, inhale deeply, and slow the pace of thoughts can regulate the nervous system and create space to sense God's presence. This is not about emptying the mind but about grounding it in truth, allowing the body's rhythms to calm as prayer and reflection settle the heart.

Physical movement also plays a vital role in reducing stress. Scripture affirms the body as a temple of the Holy Spirit, which implies care for it is an act of stewardship. Simple practices like walking, stretching, or engaging in moderate exercise can release physical tension and improve mental clarity. Combining movement with prayer or gratitude — such as taking a prayer walk — integrates body and spirit, turning ordinary activity into a moment of worship and restoration.

Another practical tool is cultivating rhythms of rest within daily life. Rest does not always mean inactivity; it is about creating intentional pauses that reset the mind and prevent burnout. These rhythms may include setting boundaries with technology, scheduling regular breaks, or building short periods of quiet reflection into the day. The Sabbath principle offers a model for this, reminding us that rest is not indulgent but commanded — a gift designed to renew strength and refocus attention on God's provision.

Engaging with Scripture in focused, meditative ways also reduces stress by reorienting thoughts toward what is true and life-giving. Passages that emphasize God's care, such as Psalm 23 or Matthew 11:28-30, can be repeated slowly in prayer, allowing the words to permeate anxious thoughts. This form of meditation shifts the focus from problems to promises, replacing worry with assurance. Over time, these practices train the mind to return to truth more readily during moments of tension.

Incorporating gratitude practices into daily routines is another way to restore calm. Gratitude shifts attention from what feels overwhelming to what is good and present, even in difficult seasons. Keeping a journal of daily blessings or pausing to thank God for three specific things each evening cultivates a posture of contentment that counters the restless nature of stress. This is not forced optimism but a conscious decision to see life through the lens of God's provision rather than lack.

Community support is equally essential for maintaining peace. Scripture emphasizes that believers are part of one body, called to bear one another's burdens. Sharing struggles with trusted friends or prayer partners not only lightens emotional load but also provides perspective that can be difficult to see alone. Encouragement from others can remind us of truths we might forget when anxiety clouds judgment. Likewise, offering support to someone else often shifts focus outward, breaking the isolation stress can create.

Establishing intentional routines helps integrate these tools into daily life rather than treating them as occasional remedies. Starting and ending the day with brief moments of stillness, Scripture, and prayer provides natural bookends that set the tone for everything in between. Regular mealtimes, consistent sleep schedules, and boundaries around work or technology help the body and mind find stability. Over time, these small acts create an environment where peace is nurtured rather than constantly disrupted.

Learning to release control into God's hands is perhaps the most transformative element of stress reduction. Many anxieties stem from trying to manage outcomes beyond our reach. Scripture repeatedly calls believers to cast their cares on God, trusting His faithfulness in both visible and unseen ways. This act of surrender does not remove responsibility for wise action, but it relieves the soul from carrying a weight it was never designed to bear.

When these practices are combined — breathing and stillness, movement, Scripture meditation, gratitude, community, and surrender — they form a holistic approach to peace that addresses body, mind, and spirit together. Stress may not vanish, but its hold weakens as the heart learns to rest in God's presence and promises. Over time, calm becomes less about escaping life's pressures and more about finding steadiness within them, anchored in the One who offers peace that the world cannot give.

Chapter 10: Community and Support in Healing

The Role of Fellowship in Biblical Healing Stories

Healing in Scripture rarely happens in isolation. While moments of private encounter with God are significant, many of the Bible's most profound healing stories occur within the context of community. Whether it is friends lowering a paralyzed man through a roof to reach Jesus, crowds gathering around Him seeking restoration, or early believers praying together for the sick, fellowship consistently serves as a channel for God's healing power. This reveals a crucial truth: relationships are not only supportive but often instrumental in the process of restoration.

The Gospels provide numerous examples of this dynamic. One of the most striking is found in Mark 2, where four friends carry a paralyzed man to Jesus. Unable to reach Him through the crowd, they climb to the roof, remove part of it, and lower their friend down to where Jesus is teaching. The text emphasizes that Jesus sees "their faith" — not only the man's — before pronouncing forgiveness and healing. This collective faith underscores the power of community intercession. The man's healing is inseparable from the commitment of those who refused to let obstacles prevent him from encountering Christ.

Fellowship also appears in stories where healing leads to restored relationships. Lepers healed by Jesus are not only freed from disease but also reinstated into the social and spiritual life of their communities. In biblical times, leprosy carried severe stigma, forcing individuals into isolation. When Jesus healed these men, the physical cure was only part of the miracle; He also restored them to belonging. This illustrates that true healing often extends beyond the body to include reintegration into fellowship, affirming dignity and connection.

The early church continued this pattern, embodying a culture where prayer, support, and shared resources fostered holistic well-being. In

Acts 2, believers are described as gathering daily, breaking bread together, and caring for each other's needs. Healing, both spiritual and physical, occurred in this context of deep relational connection. The letter of James reinforces this communal dimension by instructing believers to call the elders of the church to pray over the sick and anoint them with oil. Here, prayer for healing is not a solitary act but a family responsibility, demonstrating the importance of standing together in times of suffering.

This communal approach contrasts with modern tendencies toward individualism, where personal struggles are often hidden. Scripture offers a different vision: one in which vulnerability, prayer, and shared burdens create an environment where God's healing can flourish. Acknowledging need within fellowship does not signal weakness but reflects biblical humility and trust in God's design for His people.

Fellowship in healing also provides a safeguard against despair. When someone is physically ill or emotionally burdened, their faith may waver under the weight of exhaustion or disappointment. In those moments, the prayers and encouragement of others sustain them. The paralytic's friends in Mark 2 embody this principle, carrying him physically and spiritually when he could not carry himself. This mutual support reflects God's design for the body of Christ, where each member strengthens the others in times of weakness.

Shared healing experiences often lead to a deeper witness of God's power. When a community prays together and sees prayers answered, faith is collectively strengthened. In Acts 3, when Peter and John heal a lame man at the temple gate, the entire crowd witnesses the miracle, leading many to glorify God and listen to the gospel message. Healing becomes not only personal restoration but also a testimony that draws others to faith.

The communal aspect of healing also calls believers to active compassion. True fellowship requires more than offering words of encouragement; it involves sacrificial presence. Bearing another's burdens may mean visiting hospitals, providing meals, or sitting quietly with someone in grief. These seemingly ordinary acts become sacred when motivated by love and empowered by the Spirit. In doing so, fellowship reflects Christ Himself, who drew near to the suffering rather than avoiding them.

Modern believers can learn from these biblical examples by cultivating intentional communities where healing is nurtured. This might look like small groups committed to prayer, congregations that prioritize care ministries, or friendships built on honest sharing and mutual encouragement. The goal is not to create perfect community but to embody the kind of love Jesus described when He said the world would know His disciples by their love for one another.

Ultimately, fellowship in healing stories points to a greater reality: God designed His people not only to receive His grace individually but to reflect it collectively. When believers support, pray for, and walk alongside one another in suffering, they become living demonstrations of God's kingdom. Healing is magnified when it is shared — not simply as relief from pain, but as restoration into belonging, love, and the life of the community God has called His people to be.

How Accountability and Prayer Partners Strengthen Health

Faith was never meant to be lived in isolation. Throughout Scripture, believers are encouraged to walk together, encourage one another, and bear each other's burdens. This communal approach is not only vital for spiritual growth but also plays a significant role in emotional and physical well-being. One of the most practical expressions of this principle is found in accountability and prayer partnerships — relationships where individuals intentionally support each other in their walk with God, their struggles, and their pursuit of wholeness.

Accountability partners serve as mirrors, reflecting both progress and blind spots. Proverbs 27:17 captures this dynamic: "As iron sharpens iron, so one person sharpens another." In the context of health, this sharpening may involve gentle reminders to stay consistent with spiritual practices like prayer or fasting, encouragement to persevere in healthy habits, or honest conversations about areas where stress, bitterness, or discouragement are creeping in. Far from judgmental, this kind of accountability is rooted in love and shared commitment to growth.

Prayer partnerships take this dynamic deeper by inviting God into the process. James 5:16 instructs believers to "confess your sins to each other and pray for each other so that you may be healed." The healing described here is holistic, encompassing both spiritual and emotional restoration. Praying together creates a bond of trust and humility, allowing each person to be vulnerable about their struggles while interceding for the other. This mutual prayer strengthens faith, reminds each person they are not alone, and fosters a tangible sense of God's presence in daily life.

These partnerships also help counteract one of the greatest challenges to health in modern life: isolation. Even in a world hyperconnected by technology, many feel disconnected and unsupported. Loneliness not only affects mental health but has been linked to physical ailments, including higher risks of heart disease and weakened immunity. Accountability and prayer partners address this by offering consistent, meaningful connection. Regular check-ins, shared prayer times, and honest conversations create a sense of belonging and mutual care that directly combats the stress of isolation.

Practical benefits extend beyond emotional support. Having someone to share goals with — whether related to prayer, Scripture reading, or healthier daily rhythms — significantly increases the likelihood of follow-through. When progress is celebrated together, motivation grows; when setbacks occur, encouragement softens discouragement and helps individuals regain perspective. This steady presence can make the difference between giving up and persevering through difficult seasons.

Over time, the trust built within accountability and prayer partnerships fosters deeper transparency. As individuals share victories and failures honestly, the relationship becomes a safe space for confession and healing. This honesty breaks the isolation that often accompanies personal struggles, especially those tied to emotional burdens, unhealthy habits, or spiritual dryness. By bringing these areas into the light, the power of shame and secrecy is diminished, making room for genuine transformation.

Prayer partners also serve as reminders of God's faithfulness when personal faith feels weak. During seasons of doubt or discouragement, hearing someone else pray with conviction can rekindle hope. In this way, prayer becomes both a personal lifeline and a shared spiritual discipline, reinforcing the truth that God meets His people in community as well as individually. Mutual intercession also expands perspective; as each person prays for the other's needs, they grow in empathy and learn to see beyond their own challenges.

Consistency is what gives these partnerships lasting impact. Sporadic check-ins may encourage briefly, but intentional rhythms — whether weekly calls, in-person meetings, or daily messages — provide stability. Over time, these steady interactions shape habits of faith and resilience. They create opportunities to celebrate progress, mourn setbacks, and return continually to God's grace together. This pattern mirrors the early church, where believers devoted themselves to fellowship, prayer, and the breaking of bread as a core part of their daily lives.

The influence of such relationships often extends beyond the immediate partnership. Individuals who experience healing and growth through accountability and prayer are more likely to extend support to others, creating ripple effects within families, small groups, and congregations. This multiplication of encouragement reflects the design of the body of Christ, where each member strengthens the whole.

Ultimately, the power of accountability and prayer partners lies in their alignment with God's own method of working through relationship. Healing in Scripture is rarely solitary; it happens within families, among friends, and in the gathered church. When two believers commit to walk together with honesty and prayer, they become instruments of God's restoring work in each other's lives. Their companionship transforms struggles into opportunities for grace and provides a living testimony of what it means to bear one another's burdens and so fulfill the law of Christ.

Building a Faith-Based Support Network Today

One of the greatest resources for spiritual and emotional health is a strong community of faith. In Scripture, healing and growth often occur within the context of fellowship, where believers encourage, correct, and strengthen one another. While personal devotion and prayer are vital, the Christian life was never meant to be lived alone. Building a faith-based support network today is both a practical and spiritual endeavor, providing an anchor in seasons of struggle and a source of joy in seasons of celebration.

A support network begins with intentional relationships. In a culture that prizes independence, forming these connections may require deliberate effort. Start by identifying those who share a desire to grow spiritually and value authenticity. These might be members of a church, a small group, or even friends met through service or study gatherings. The quality of the connection matters more than the size; a small circle of trusted companions often provides deeper support than a large network of acquaintances.

Shared faith forms the foundation for this network. Believers are united not by common interests alone but by a commitment to follow Christ together. This shared commitment creates space for mutual encouragement and accountability rooted in Scripture rather than personal opinion. It also allows for prayer that is specific and Spirit-led, addressing needs with confidence in God's promises. When life's challenges arise, knowing others are interceding provides tangible comfort and strengthens personal trust in God's care.

Diversity within the network enriches its impact. Including people of different ages, experiences, and spiritual gifts offers varied perspectives and wisdom. Older believers can provide guidance drawn from years of walking with God, while peers can offer empathy through shared life stages. This intergenerational dynamic reflects the New Testament model of the church as a family, where everyone contributes and everyone benefits.

The strength of a faith-based support network also depends on its depth. True support is built on honesty and vulnerability. This requires creating an environment where struggles can be shared without fear of judgment. Building such trust takes time and intentionality: listening well, keeping confidences, and extending grace. Over time, this culture of openness becomes a safe place for confession, healing, and growth.

Regular rhythms of connection are essential to keeping the network strong. Without consistent interaction, relationships can become superficial and lose their ability to provide meaningful support. Scheduling weekly or biweekly meetings, whether in person or online, helps maintain momentum. These gatherings do not need to be elaborate; even simple check-ins that include prayer, Scripture reflection, and honest sharing can foster significant growth and encouragement over time.

Serving together further deepens bonds. When members of a faith-based network join efforts to meet the needs of others — volunteering at a local shelter, supporting missions, or caring for someone within the group — they experience unity in action. Shared service shifts the focus from individual struggles to collective purpose, reminding everyone of the bigger story God is writing through their lives. This outward orientation strengthens fellowship and cultivates humility, compassion, and joy.

Healthy boundaries play an important role in sustaining supportive networks. While deep sharing is vital, members must respect each other's capacity and privacy. Support should never feel like control or intrusion. Instead, the aim is to encourage without pressuring and to offer help without fostering dependency. When handled with grace, these boundaries create space for authentic care without burdening any one person with unrealistic expectations.

Over time, the impact of such a network becomes evident not only in spiritual growth but also in emotional resilience and physical well-being. Studies consistently show that strong social connections contribute to lower stress, improved mental health, and even better physical outcomes during illness. Scripture affirms this reality, calling believers to "encourage one another and build each other up" (1 Thessalonians 5:11). In living this out, a faith-based support network becomes more than a group of friends; it becomes an expression of the body of Christ, where each member helps the others flourish.

The ultimate goal of building and sustaining these relationships is mutual transformation. As members walk through life together — celebrating answered prayers, grieving losses, confessing sins, and rejoicing in growth — they become living witnesses of God's faithfulness. The network itself becomes a testimony to the power of fellowship rooted in Christ, offering a tangible example of the healing and wholeness that arise when believers choose to journey together in love and truth.

Part IV. Walking Forward in God's Healing Plan

Reaching a place of healing is not the end of the journey; it is the beginning of a new way of living. The principles explored so far — forgiveness, trust, community, prayer, and aligning with God's design — are not simply ideas to visit once but foundations for a lifestyle. Walking forward in God's healing plan means choosing daily to remain rooted in His presence, to nurture what He has restored, and to grow in maturity as challenges inevitably arise.

This stage of the journey is about integration. Healing that stays abstract or theoretical fades quickly under the weight of life's pressures. But healing that becomes habit — woven into thought patterns, daily rhythms, and responses to stress — endures. Scripture describes this process not as a moment but as a walk, a continual movement toward wholeness guided by the Spirit. As Paul writes in Galatians 5, walking by the Spirit leads to fruit that cannot be manufactured: love, joy, peace, patience, kindness, and self-control. These qualities become evidence of the inner transformation God has brought about.

Walking forward also requires vigilance. The world around us remains chaotic, full of noise, distraction, and pressures that can pull the heart away from peace. Old wounds may resurface, temptations may reappear, and discouragement may whisper that progress is temporary. God's healing plan does not promise a life free from struggle, but it does promise His presence and power to meet each challenge. Remaining anchored in prayer, Scripture, and fellowship equips believers to navigate these seasons with renewed strength.

This part of the book is designed to move from reflection to practice. It will explore how to live out healing in everyday contexts: in relationships, in personal habits, and in responding to life's inevitable changes. It will look at sustaining inner peace, sharing what God has done with others, and embracing the calling that comes with restored wholeness.

Ultimately, this walk is not just about personal well-being but about becoming a conduit of healing for others — carrying forward the love and grace that have been received into every sphere of life.

Chapter 11: Integrating Body, Mind, and Spirit

Holistic Healing in Scripture: Not Just Physical Health

When most people think of healing, physical recovery is often the first image that comes to mind. In Scripture, however, healing is rarely limited to the body. The Bible presents a broader, richer vision — one where restoration touches every part of a person's life: mind, emotions, relationships, and spirit. This holistic perspective reveals that God's desire for His people is not merely the absence of illness but the presence of wholeness.

From the earliest pages of Genesis, human beings are depicted as integrated creations. The body, soul, and spirit are not separate compartments but interwoven dimensions of one life. What affects the body influences the mind and spirit; what burdens the soul often manifests physically. Modern research affirms this interconnectedness, showing how emotional stress impacts immunity or how unresolved trauma affects long-term health. Scripture anticipated this truth long before it was studied in laboratories, consistently addressing people as whole beings rather than disjointed parts.

The ministry of Jesus offers vivid illustrations of this holistic approach. When He healed, He often addressed more than physical symptoms. To the paralyzed man lowered through the roof in Mark 2, Jesus first said, "Your sins are forgiven," before telling him to rise and walk. This order reveals something profound: inner restoration was as essential as outward mobility. For the woman with the issue of blood, healing included both the cessation of bleeding and the public affirmation of her dignity, restoring her to community after years of isolation.

Holistic healing in Scripture also involves the renewal of relationships. Sin, brokenness, and illness often fracture connections — with God, with others, and even with oneself. When God brings healing, He restores harmony to these relationships. Zacchaeus, after encountering Christ, not only experienced personal transformation but also sought to make restitution to those he had wronged. His healing was social and spiritual as well as internal, demonstrating that God's work always moves outward into the broader fabric of life.

This vision of wholeness challenges modern tendencies to treat symptoms rather than root causes. It invites believers to consider whether stress, bitterness, fear, or unforgiveness may underlie persistent struggles. Healing, according to Scripture, often begins in the heart — addressing what cannot be seen but profoundly shapes what is felt and lived. This is why practices like confession, forgiveness, gratitude, and worship are central to biblical healing. They open the door for God's Spirit to restore what no physical remedy alone can reach.

Holistic healing also speaks to the restoration of purpose. Illness and brokenness often strip life of meaning, leaving individuals feeling disconnected from their calling. In Scripture, when God restores someone, He often reorients them toward mission. Peter's reinstatement after denying Christ is one example: Jesus not only forgives him but commissions him to "feed My sheep." Healing becomes the foundation for service, transforming personal restoration into blessing for others.

The Psalms demonstrate how emotional and spiritual renewal are integral to health. David's prayers frequently move from lament to praise, showing a shift in focus from pain to trust. This process of pouring out fears and receiving God's peace highlights the connection between emotional honesty and spiritual resilience. Modern studies on gratitude and mindfulness confirm what the Psalms have modeled for centuries — that turning attention to God's faithfulness calms the nervous system and fosters deeper well-being.

Communal elements are central to this vision of healing. The early church in Acts exemplifies a community where physical needs, spiritual growth, and emotional support were addressed together. Believers shared meals, prayed for one another, and cared for the poor in a rhythm of life that reflected God's kingdom. This interconnected care was not an optional supplement to personal faith but a core expression of discipleship. Healing in this context was not just about individuals but about the restoration of an entire people shaped by God's love.

Holistic healing also acknowledges the tension between the "already" and "not yet" of God's kingdom. While believers may experience profound restoration in this life, full healing will only be complete in the presence of God. This perspective fosters both hope and humility: hope that God is actively redeeming what is broken, and humility to trust Him even when healing unfolds slowly or differently than expected. Such trust allows believers to seek wholeness without demanding perfection, resting in God's promise to make all things new.

Embracing this biblical vision invites a shift in how health is pursued today. Rather than separating physical care from spiritual life, it calls for integration — nourishing the body through wise choices, the mind through renewed thoughts, and the spirit through prayer and worship. It also encourages addressing relational wounds, practicing forgiveness, and seeking community as part of the healing process. In doing so, believers align with God's holistic design, experiencing peace that goes beyond the absence of illness and enters into the fullness of life He intends.

The Interplay of Thoughts, Emotions, and Spiritual Life

Scripture consistently recognizes the deep connection between what we think, what we feel, and how we live before God. Modern science confirms this, showing that thoughts and emotions influence physical health, decision-making, and relational patterns. Yet the Bible revealed this integration long before neuroscience existed, offering a blueprint for transforming the mind and spirit together. Understanding this interplay is essential for those seeking lasting healing and peace.

The mind serves as a gateway to the heart. Proverbs 4:23 urges believers to guard their hearts, "for everything you do flows from it," yet it is often through thoughts that the heart is shaped. Repeated thought patterns create emotional responses, which in turn guide behavior. For example, dwelling on fear cultivates anxiety, which affects both mood and physical well-being. Conversely, meditating on God's promises fosters trust and hope, leading to resilience even amid trials.

Paul's instruction in Romans 12:2 to "be transformed by the renewing of your mind" highlights this principle. Transformation begins internally, with the reshaping of thought life according to God's truth. This renewal is not about ignoring reality but reframing it. Difficult circumstances are acknowledged, yet they are viewed through the lens of God's sovereignty and faithfulness. Over time, this shift in perspective reshapes emotions, softening despair into hope and anger into compassion.

Emotions, in turn, are not enemies to be suppressed but signals to be understood. The Psalms are filled with raw emotion — joy, sorrow, anger, fear — yet these emotions are continually brought before God in prayer. This honesty fosters intimacy with Him and prevents unprocessed feelings from hardening into bitterness or despair. In this sense, emotional health is not found in pretending everything is fine but in learning to meet God honestly in the midst of life's complexities.

The spiritual life both influences and is influenced by thoughts and emotions. Times of spiritual dryness often coincide with negative thought patterns or emotional fatigue, while seasons of vibrant faith are marked by renewed mental focus and inner peace. Practices like Scripture meditation, prayer, and worship serve as recalibrating forces, realigning the mind and heart toward God's presence. These disciplines not only draw believers closer to Him but also strengthen emotional stability and mental clarity.

When thoughts are aligned with God's truth, emotions gradually follow suit. This alignment does not erase difficulty but equips believers to navigate it differently. Fear gives way to courage when anchored in promises of God's protection. Guilt yields to gratitude when grace is fully grasped. Even grief, while still painful, becomes infused with hope when framed by the assurance of resurrection and eternal life. This transformation is subtle and ongoing, requiring repeated return to Scripture and prayer rather than a single moment of resolve.

The practice of taking thoughts captive, as Paul describes in 2 Corinthians 10:5, illustrates a proactive approach. Instead of allowing harmful narratives to run unchecked — thoughts of unworthiness, hopelessness, or resentment — believers are called to measure every idea against the truth of Christ. This intentional filtering reshapes emotional responses over time. It does not mean ignoring difficult realities but reframing them with the awareness that God is present and at work, even in hardship.

Healthy emotions can also deepen spiritual life. Compassion, for example, often fuels intercessory prayer and acts of service. Joy inspires worship that goes beyond obligation into genuine delight. Even lament, when directed toward God, becomes a pathway to intimacy, as seen in the psalms where grief turns to praise within the same prayer. Rather than being a hindrance to faith, emotions become vehicles through which believers experience God's presence more fully.

Holistic healing emerges when mind, heart, and spirit work in harmony. This integration allows believers to live authentically — acknowledging pain without being ruled by it, celebrating blessings without clinging to them, and trusting God's goodness in both abundance and scarcity. Over time, this wholeness creates stability that is not dependent on external circumstances. It is rooted in an inner life formed by truth and sustained by the Spirit's presence.

Cultivating this harmony requires intentional practices woven into daily life. Regular Scripture reading trains the mind in truth. Honest prayer gives voice to emotions and invites God into them. Fellowship provides perspective and encouragement, preventing isolation that often distorts thoughts and intensifies negative emotions. Together, these rhythms build resilience and nurture peace that endures beyond momentary feelings.

The interplay of thoughts, emotions, and spiritual life reveals that healing is not merely about fixing one part of the self but restoring the whole person. As believers learn to surrender both their inner narratives and their deepest feelings to God, they discover freedom and stability that flow into every aspect of life. This is the kind of healing Scripture envisions — a transformation that touches mind, heart, and soul, drawing the entire person into deeper communion with the One who created them.

Creating a Personal Healing Framework Anchored in Faith

Healing that lasts rarely happens by accident. It grows out of intentional choices, daily rhythms, and a clear understanding of what anchors the process. Scripture provides not only the principles of healing but also the foundation for building a framework that integrates body, mind, and spirit in alignment with God's design. This framework is deeply personal — shaped by each individual's circumstances, strengths, and struggles — yet rooted in timeless truths that apply to all who seek wholeness in Christ.

The first step in creating such a framework is recognizing that healing is holistic. Physical health cannot be separated from emotional well-being or spiritual vitality. A person may improve their diet, exercise regularly, and still feel restless if bitterness remains unresolved or if they lack connection with God. Similarly, focusing on prayer while neglecting rest, nourishment, or relationships can lead to imbalance. Scripture invites believers to view life as an integrated whole, where each aspect affects the others and contributes to overall flourishing.

Building on this understanding begins with identifying what areas of life need renewal. Honest reflection is key: Are stress and anxiety undermining physical health? Are unhealthy relationships draining emotional reserves? Has spiritual life grown dry, leaving the heart distant from God? Taking inventory in prayer allows believers to invite God into every part of their story, acknowledging the places where His healing is most needed. This openness becomes the foundation for lasting transformation.

Once areas of need are recognized, the next step is establishing practices that nurture alignment with God's design. Scripture and prayer remain central, not only as sources of comfort but as guides for perspective and action. Meditating on passages about God's care, such as Psalm 23 or Matthew 11:28-30, shifts focus from fear to trust. Regular prayer — both personal and in community — invites the Holy Spirit to transform thoughts and emotions, strengthening faith during the ups and downs of the healing process.

Practical steps also play a crucial role in sustaining this framework. Setting rhythms of rest and work, prioritizing nourishing foods, incorporating movement, and cultivating gratitude create an environment where healing can take root. These choices, though small on their own, accumulate into patterns that reinforce physical and emotional stability. When rooted in faith, even ordinary routines become acts of worship, reminding believers that caring for the body and soul honors the One who created them.

Accountability strengthens this framework, ensuring that commitments are more than good intentions. Sharing goals with a trusted friend, mentor, or prayer partner creates space for encouragement and honest reflection. This support helps maintain consistency when motivation wanes and offers perspective when progress feels slow. In biblical community, growth is celebrated together, and setbacks are met with grace rather than shame. This mirrors the pattern seen in the early church, where believers were strengthened by prayer and mutual care.

Flexibility is equally important. A healing framework is not a rigid checklist but a living guide that adjusts as circumstances change. Life seasons vary — times of rest, transition, or crisis each bring unique demands. Anchoring the framework in God's unchanging truth allows for this adaptability without losing focus. Practices may shift in form, but their purpose remains constant: staying aligned with God's presence and design for wholeness.

Surrender forms the core of this entire process. Without yielding control to God, even the best intentions can become exhausting attempts to fix oneself. Healing anchored in faith acknowledges dependence on Him, trusting that His wisdom surpasses personal understanding. This surrender is not passive resignation but active trust, inviting God into every decision, emotion, and step forward. It is the posture Jesus modeled in Gethsemane, choosing the Father's will even when the path was difficult.

As the framework takes shape and becomes part of daily life, healing begins to extend outward. Inner peace fosters healthier relationships, renewed energy inspires service, and spiritual growth equips believers to encourage others on their own journeys. Personal wholeness becomes a testimony, pointing to the God who restores not only individuals but entire communities. This ripple effect reflects the heart of biblical healing — transformation that begins within and spreads outward, glorifying God in every sphere of life.

In the end, creating a personal healing framework is less about constructing a perfect system and more about cultivating a way of life rooted in God's presence. It is about walking with Him in the ordinary moments, trusting His guidance through challenges, and allowing His Spirit to integrate every part of life into a unified pursuit of wholeness. This kind of framework does not eliminate struggle, but it ensures that even in difficulty, believers remain grounded, purposeful, and anchored in the One who promises to make all things new.

Chapter 12: Walking Forward in God's Healing Plan

Living Daily in Alignment with Scripture

Living in alignment with Scripture is not about adding another task to an already crowded schedule but about allowing God's Word to shape every aspect of life. This alignment turns biblical truth from something read occasionally into something lived continuously, influencing thoughts, emotions, relationships, and decisions. It transforms healing from a momentary experience into a sustained way of being.

The process begins with intimacy. Scripture is not meant to be approached as a mere textbook of rules but as a personal letter from God, revealing His character and inviting relationship. When believers read the Word seeking to know Him, rather than just to gather information, the text becomes alive. Verses move from abstract ideas to personal guidance, offering direction in decisions and reassurance in moments of uncertainty. This intimacy shifts Scripture from obligation to desire — from something to check off to something that nourishes.

Integrating Scripture into daily life requires consistency. Short bursts of inspiration, while helpful, cannot replace steady exposure to God's truth. Just as the body thrives on regular nourishment rather than occasional feasts, the spirit needs ongoing engagement with the Word. This may look like structured reading plans, meditation on a single verse throughout the day, or journaling prayers in response to what God is revealing. The goal is not speed or volume but depth — allowing the Word to sink in and transform.

Alignment with Scripture also involves obedience. Understanding God's Word is incomplete if it remains theoretical. Healing and transformation occur when knowledge is translated into action. Forgiveness must be extended, even when difficult. Trust must be practiced, even when circumstances are uncertain. Generosity, humility, and compassion must move beyond admiration into daily choices. Each small act of obedience becomes a building block for a life that reflects God's design and fosters lasting peace.

A crucial element of this alignment is discernment. In a world flooded with voices — cultural pressures, personal desires, and conflicting opinions — Scripture serves as the standard by which all is measured. This discernment helps believers navigate decisions about health, relationships, work, and personal growth without being swayed by every new trend or fear. It grounds them in unchanging truth, providing clarity amid confusion and stability amid chaos.

Living out Scripture daily also cultivates resilience during hardship. When trials arise, those who have built their lives around God's Word draw on a deep well of truth rather than scrambling for comfort. Familiar passages come to mind in moments of fear, guiding responses and renewing strength. This is what Jesus demonstrated during His temptation in the wilderness, countering lies with Scripture He had internalized. Such resilience does not remove struggle but equips believers to face it anchored in something greater than circumstances.

Community enhances this alignment. Scripture was given not only to individuals but to the body of Christ. Engaging with the Word in fellowship — through study groups, shared prayer, or even simple conversations — adds layers of understanding and accountability. Others may highlight insights missed in solitary reading, and mutual encouragement fosters perseverance when personal resolve wanes. This shared pursuit creates a culture where living by Scripture becomes a collective norm rather than an isolated effort.

Reflection is another key practice. Without pausing to examine how Scripture intersects with daily life, it is easy to drift into routine. Regular self-examination — asking where one's thoughts, habits, and relationships align with or diverge from God's Word — opens space for continual growth. This reflection is not about condemnation but about inviting God to gently correct and redirect. Over time, it fosters humility and a willingness to be shaped, ensuring that faith remains dynamic rather than stagnant.

The fruit of living in alignment with Scripture becomes evident not only internally but outwardly. Peace replaces anxiety, patience softens irritability, and compassion overflows into relationships. These qualities are not manufactured by effort alone but produced as the Spirit works through surrendered hearts. Others notice the difference, often long before the individual does, and this quiet witness points people toward Christ more powerfully than words alone ever could.

Ultimately, aligning life with Scripture is about abiding — remaining connected to the source of wisdom, comfort, and truth. It is a continual returning, a daily decision to let God's voice be louder than every other influence. This abiding transforms not just moments of crisis but the ordinary rhythms of life: how one speaks, responds, prioritizes, and serves. It is here that healing deepens, taking root beyond surface habits into the core of identity, shaping a life that reflects the heart of God in every season.

Avoiding Extremes: Faith and Wisdom in Balance

Scripture calls believers to live by faith, trusting God's promises even when circumstances seem uncertain. At the same time, it commends wisdom — careful discernment, stewardship, and planning that honors God's design for life. Holding these two together can be challenging. Some lean toward extreme reliance on personal understanding, sidelining faith in favor of control. Others swing toward presumption, expecting God to act without engaging in wise decisions or practical responsibility. Both extremes can hinder healing and spiritual growth.

Biblical faith is never blind recklessness. Hebrews 11 celebrates those who trusted God in radical ways, but their faith was rooted in His character, not in careless optimism. Noah built the ark in response to God's specific warning. Abraham left his homeland because God called him to a new land. Their faith was active — not passive waiting, but obedient steps taken in response to God's guidance. This model demonstrates that faith involves trust paired with action, rather than ignoring practical considerations.

Wisdom, likewise, is celebrated throughout Scripture as a divine gift. Proverbs portrays wisdom as essential for navigating daily life, guarding against harm, and fostering peace. It teaches prudence in speech, moderation in habits, and diligence in work. James 1:5 encourages believers to ask God for wisdom, promising that He gives generously to those who seek it. Wisdom does not compete with faith; it complements it. Faith provides the courage to act, while wisdom guides how and when to act.

Tension arises when believers misunderstand the relationship between these two virtues. Relying on faith alone without seeking wisdom can lead to avoidable harm — neglecting rest, refusing medical help, or making impulsive decisions under the banner of trust. Conversely, clinging to human wisdom without faith can result in anxiety, overcontrol, and resistance to God's leading. The healthiest path is found where trust in God's sovereignty and commitment to wise living meet.

This balance is particularly relevant in the context of healing. A person may pray for recovery while also pursuing medical treatment, seeking counsel, or adjusting lifestyle habits. Trusting God for provision does not negate budgeting wisely or working diligently. Seeking peace in relationships involves prayer for reconciliation as well as humble conversations and practical boundaries. In each case, faith and wisdom work together rather than in isolation.

Walking in this balance begins with humility. Faith recognizes that God's ways are higher than human understanding, while wisdom acknowledges the need to discern and apply those ways thoughtfully. Humility prevents the arrogance of assuming every decision must rely solely on personal logic, and it also guards against the presumption that God will always override poor choices. This posture allows believers to seek His will earnestly, using both prayer and practical insight as tools for discernment.

Jesus Himself modeled this harmony. He trusted the Father completely yet made careful decisions in ministry — withdrawing to pray, avoiding premature confrontation, and providing practical care for the hungry crowds. His life demonstrates that deep faith and sound judgment are not opposites but partners. Following His example, believers are called to listen for God's voice while also using the wisdom He provides through Scripture, counsel, and experience.

Practically, balancing faith and wisdom means examining motives and outcomes. Are decisions motivated by fear disguised as caution, or by recklessness labeled as trust? Are choices leading toward peace, love, and greater reliance on God, or do they result in confusion and harm? These questions invite honest reflection and ensure actions are guided by both prayerful dependence and thoughtful evaluation.

In the context of healing, this balance fosters sustainable growth. Trust in God's power encourages hope when progress is slow, while wisdom informs healthy habits that support recovery. Someone seeking emotional restoration may combine prayer with counseling or journaling. A believer desiring physical healing might pray for strength while making changes to rest, diet, and stress management. Faith fuels perseverance; wisdom shapes the path forward.

Living in this tension also prepares believers for seasons of uncertainty. There will be moments when God's leading defies conventional logic, requiring bold trust. There will also be times when His answer comes through practical solutions or gradual change rather than immediate intervention. Holding both realities allows believers to remain steady, avoiding despair when miracles do not come instantly and resisting pride when blessings unfold through ordinary means.

Ultimately, faith and wisdom together create a life anchored in God's character and guided by His Spirit. This balance produces resilience, discernment, and peace, enabling believers to navigate challenges with confidence that God is present in both the miraculous and the mundane. It is here, in the quiet convergence of trust and prudence, that true healing and wholeness are sustained.

Continuing the Journey: Growth, Maintenance, and Hope

Healing is not a single event but a lifelong process. Even after significant breakthroughs, the journey continues, requiring ongoing care, intentional practices, and a vision for what lies ahead. Scripture portrays this reality often: God delivers His people, but He also calls them to walk faithfully afterward. The exodus from Egypt was followed by a wilderness journey, and the early church's initial outpouring of the Spirit was followed by decades of perseverance and discipleship. In the same way, personal healing begins a new chapter rather than concluding the story.

Growth in this stage is often quieter but no less profound. While initial seasons of healing can feel dramatic, ongoing transformation tends to happen through steady rhythms rather than sudden shifts. Faithful prayer, Scripture meditation, and community support create an environment where the roots of healing sink deeper. These practices turn lessons learned into lasting character, preventing old wounds from reopening when life becomes stressful or uncertain.

Maintenance involves recognizing potential triggers and addressing them with wisdom rather than fear. Past patterns may resurface in subtle ways, especially during times of fatigue, transition, or disappointment. This is not failure but an invitation to apply what has been learned. Staying grounded in God's promises helps believers respond with resilience rather than panic. Psalm 1 paints a picture of this stability, describing the righteous as trees planted by streams of water, bearing fruit in every season because their roots remain nourished.

Hope sustains the journey when progress feels slow. Healing often unfolds in layers, revealing deeper areas for growth over time. Each step forward, no matter how small, is a sign of God's ongoing work. Hope looks ahead, trusting that the same God who began the process will continue it to completion. This confidence does not deny challenges but places them within the larger story of redemption, where ultimate restoration awaits in God's presence.

As the journey continues, intentional reflection becomes essential. Taking time to look back on how far God has brought you fosters gratitude and guards against complacency. Remembering answered prayers and milestones of growth provides perspective when current struggles feel overwhelming. In the Old Testament, God often instructed His people to build memorials or altars after significant events, not only to honor Him but to remind future generations of His faithfulness. Creating personal reminders — journaling, marking dates, or sharing testimonies — serves a similar purpose today.

Remaining open to further growth keeps the heart soft and responsive to God's leading. Healing does not mean every question is answered or every challenge resolved. Life will present new seasons, each revealing fresh opportunities for trust and deeper surrender. Rather than fearing this ongoing process, believers can embrace it as evidence of God's active presence. Spiritual maturity is not a destination to arrive at but a continual becoming — being shaped more fully into the likeness of Christ.

Community continues to play a vital role in this stage. Support networks that were helpful in early healing remain just as important for maintaining it. Walking with others in faith ensures accountability and encouragement, especially during times when old habits threaten to resurface. In turn, those who have experienced restoration often find themselves equipped to help others on their own journeys. This outward focus not only blesses others but reinforces personal growth, turning pain into purpose.

Anchoring daily life in hope also changes how believers face setbacks. When challenges come — whether new hardships or echoes of past wounds — hope reminds them that God's story is not finished. This forward-looking faith transforms how difficulties are perceived, shifting them from obstacles to opportunities for reliance on Him. Paul captured this perspective in Philippians 3, urging believers to forget what is behind and press forward toward what lies ahead.

Ultimately, growth, maintenance, and hope form a cycle rather than a straight line. Healing deepens through rhythms of reflection, adaptation, and renewed trust. Over time, this ongoing journey shapes a life that is both resilient and tender, grounded yet open to God's future work. It becomes a living testimony that healing is not a single moment but a lifelong invitation to walk closely with the One who restores all things.

Last Words: Thank You

If you have reached this page, it means you have taken the time to walk through these pages with an open heart and a searching spirit. That is no small thing. In a world filled with noise and distraction, choosing to slow down and seek truth is an act of courage. For that, I want to say thank you.

Thank you for trusting me enough to explore these teachings. Thank you for being willing to look deeper into Scripture, not just as a historical text, but as a living invitation to healing and restoration. Thank you for opening yourself to practices that, while ancient, still speak life into our modern struggles.

This journey is not meant to end here. My hope is that what you have read will stay with you — that these truths will guide your decisions, comfort you in moments of doubt, and remind you that healing is possible even in the hardest seasons. May the seeds planted in these chapters grow into something enduring and beautiful in your life.

I also want to encourage you to share what you have found. Healing is multiplied when it is passed on. Whether through a kind word, a prayer, or simply living with renewed peace, your life can be a light to others who are searching.

Above all, remember this: you are not forgotten, you are not alone, and you are deeply loved by the One who made you. May His presence guide you, sustain you, and bring you peace as you continue forward.

Thank you for letting me be part of your story.

www.ingramcontent.com/pod-product-compliance
Lightning Source LLC
Chambersburg PA
CBHW070252290326
41930CB00041B/2456